SEX EDUCATION AND COUNSELLING
FOR MENTALLY HANDICAPPED PEOPLE

Sex Education & Counseling for Mentally Handicapped People

ANN CRAFT
AND
MICHAEL CRAFT

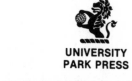

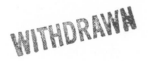

**UNIVERSITY
PARK PRESS**

UNIVERSITY PARK PRESS

BALTIMORE

UNIVERSITY PARK PRESS

Published in the United States of America
in 1983 by University Park Press,
300 North Charles Street, Baltimore, Maryland 21201

Copyright © Ann and Michael Craft
ISBN 0 8391 1773 6
Library of Congress Catalogue Number 82 50831

Printed by The Pitman Press, Lower Bristol Road,
Bath BA2 3BL

Contents

Foreword	*Sol Gordon*	vii
List of Contributors		ix
Preface	*Stanley Segal*	xiii
1. Sexuality and Mental Retardation: a review of the literature	*Ann Craft*	1
2. Sexual Behaviour and Sexual Difficulties	*Michael Craft*	38
3. Sexuality Training for Professionals who work with Mentally Handicapped Persons	*Winifred Kempton*	53
4. Counselling Parents and Care Staff on the Sexual Needs of Mentally Handicapped People	*Winifred Kempton and Frank Caparulo*	78
5. The Parents' Viewpoint	*Pauline Fairbrother*	95
6. Health, Sex and Hygiene Education in Special Schools	*June McNaughton*	110
7. Why is it such a Big Secret? Sex Education for Handicapped Young Adults	*Hilary Brown*	131
8. A Health and Sex Education Programme: Curriculum and Resources	*Ann Craft, Jean Davis Maldwyn Williams and Marjorie Williams*	148
9. Teaching Programmes and Training Techniques	*Ann Craft*	186
10. Sexuality in the Ongoing Lives of Mildly Retarded Adults	*Paul Koegel and Robert Whittemore*	213
11. Birth Control Techniques and Counselling for a Mentally Handicapped Population	*Rona MacLean*	241
12. Sexuality Counselling with Developmentally Disabled Couples	*Linda Andron*	254
13. An International Perspective	*Victoria Shennan*	287
14. Implications for the Future	*Ann and Michael Craft*	299
Index		305

Foreword

We have finally reached the point where both professionals and parents believe it's urgent to meet the sexual needs of mentally handicapped people. Both research and clinical evidence are clear: without knowledge and understanding, mentally handicapped individuals suffer. This book is warmly welcome for bringing together with an international perspective some of the outstanding thinkers and humanists in the field. With careful attention to research and a thorough review of the literature, we have available for the first time, for the American and British professional, the rich body of material that has been developed.

No book that I know of makes so clear the direction we must take in terms of counselling, birth control techniques and the special role in training professional and paraprofessional staff who work with those who are mentally handicapped. Such vital issues as marriage, reproduction, institutional policies, sterilization and consent from the developmentally handicapped themselves for surgical procedures are covered thoroughly. This volume provides numerous practical suggestions for implementing seminars and workshops designed for training staff and key personnel.

A special feature throughout the writers' contributions is a sensitive treatment of the attitudes that professionals bring to their work with mentally handicapped people that both impede and enhance the development of their clients. Our profession can only be grateful to the Crafts for their contribution in bringing together in one volume an outstanding representative group of experts.

Sol Gordon, Ph.D.
Professor, Department of Child and
Family Studies, Syracuse University

List of Contributors

LINDA ANDRON has a master's degree in social work. She has a special interest in sexual counselling, particularly with developmentally delayed clients. She has pioneered investigations and treatment of sexual dysfunction among this population and is the author of several articles on the subject.

HILARY BROWN is a qualified teacher, experienced in working with mentally handicapped people in a variety of residential settings, both in the UK and USA. She is Head of Living Skills at the Spastics Society's Dene College and has developed personal and social skills programmes, including sex education courses, for the multiply handicapped young residential students. She has just completed an M.Sc. in Health Education.

FRANK CAPARULO has much experience in the field of health and sex education and serves on the Board of the Sex Information and Education Council of the United States. He is a Family Counsellor in Connecticut, and is the author of a number of publications concerning human sexuality.

ANN CRAFT is a research social worker at Bryn y Neuadd Hospital. She was joint recipient (with Michael Craft) of a grant to investigate mentally handicapped married couples within Wales. She has developed audiovisual health and sex education teaching material for mentally handicapped audiences, and is involved in the counselling service run by the hospital for single, engaged and married mentally handicapped residents.

MICHAEL CRAFT is a consultant psychiatrist, specialising in mental handicap. He graduated in neurology at Edinburgh University and studied psychiatry at the Maudsley Hospital, London. He evolved guardianship and boarding out systems for long stay hospital residents with local authorities, social service departments, and developed a forensic psychiatric service with probation officers in Wales. He has recently edited the 12th edition of *Tredgold's Mental Retardation*.

JEAN DAVIS currently works as a speech therapy aide at Bryn y Neuadd Hospital. Previously she was a nursing assistant, and has worked in mental handicap hospitals for twenty years. She is part of the Bryn y Neuadd counselling team.

PAULINE FAIRBROTHER is the mother of a mentally handicapped daughter and has been active in improving the rights of mentally handicapped people for many years. She is a member of the National Council of the Royal Society for Mentally Handicapped Children and Adults.

WINIFRED KEMPTON is a leading authority on sexuality and mental handicap, and is the author of key books in the field. She lectures extensively both in the USA and elsewhere, and has run numerous training workshops on sexuality for parents and care-workers. She is consultant in training and socialization of disabled persons to the Planned Parenthood of Southeastern Pennsylvania.

PAUL KOEGEL is an anthropologist with the Socio-Behavioral Group of the Mental Retardation Research Center, University of California, Los Angeles. His work has centred on the community adaptation of mildly retarded individuals, with special focus on such areas as socialized incompetence, sexuality, employment, social support systems, and retardation in the black community. Outside of the field of mental retardation, his interests lie in medical anthropology and the study of deviance in cross-cultural perspective.

RONA MACLEAN is a psychiatrist. After qualifying she worked for some time in obstetrics and gynaecology and became interested in the psychosomatic aspects of the specialities. This led to a formal training in psychiatry and eventually to a consultant appointment in the field of mental handicap at the Manor Hospital, Epsom, where she also runs a Family Planning Clinic.

JUNE MCNAUGHTON was formerly Head of the Remedial Department in an Essex Comprehensive School and also taught in Special Schools before a post as the Project Officer with the Schools Council, producing health education teaching materials for slow learners. Currently she is Director of Health Education for Slow Learners for a three-year programme based at Bath University.

VICTORIA SHENNAN has served the Royal Society for Mentally Handicapped Children and Adults for the past twelve years as Publications Director. She has worked as a tutor in Health Education in the UK and the Caribbean where she wrote a course in Health Education for Rural Schools for the Ministry of Education, Jamaica. She has lectured in several countries and is the author of a number of books and articles on mental handicap, the latest being concerned with homes in the community for retarded people.

ROBERT D. WHITTEMORE, an anthropologist, has largely concerned himself with the socialisation of both normal and mentally retarded individuals. His research with the mildly retarded has focussed on sexuality, the role of siblings in the developing lives of the retarded, and the issue of adaptive competence. He is currently conducting research among the Mandinka in West Africa on changing patterns of work within the African family and their effect on children's social development.

MALDWYN WILLIAMS is a qualified teacher and has been the Adult Education Officer at Bryn y Neuadd Hospital for the past nine years. He is a member of the hospital's counselling team.

MARJORIE WILLIAMS is a nursing assistant at Bryn y Neuadd Hospital. She runs the hospital's Domestic Training Unit which teaches homecraft skills to residents, and is a member of the counselling team.

Preface

Stanley Segal

The concept of 'sex education' prompts complex reactions and contradictory attitudes even when the recipients of the education are of normal ability. An issue of the *Times Educational Supplement*—current at the time of writing—includes a report stating that at the Government's insistence, material for the Health Educational Council's new sex education campaign has been personally vetted by ministers from the Departments of Health and Education. The report refers also to the fact that the Council has run into trouble with previous campaigns. Cinema managers once refused to show a film intended for young people with anything other than an X certificate adults-only programme, while advertisements in another press campaign concerned with contraception were refused by the *Sun* and *Daily Mirror* (*TES* 8/1/82).

Adding the term 'mental handicap' to 'sex education' stirs even more conflicting emotions. We are, after all, considering persons with a wide range of mental and physical abilities, many of whom stand on the borders of classification and might be assessed differently in different countries. However, the decade which began with the United Nations Declaration of the Rights of the Mentally Handicapped (1971) was marked by the increasing impetus of two separate, but linked, movements with roots in the 1960s. One was the shift in public attitudes towards open discussion and consideration of sexual matters; the other movement has proclaimed the rights of various disadvantaged groups in society to as normal a life as possible. These rights were seen by many to include social and educational integration and sexual expression.

Within our context of mental handicap the question then arises: how can pupils, staff, parents and allied professionals best be prepared for this changing context which has as its aim an improvement in the quality of life for individuals who are handicapped? Books and articles opened up debate and discussion, carried on in conferences and workshops on both sides of the Atlantic. But the new drive not only brought greater opportunities, but greater risks. Solutions of problems connected with greater integration of 'the handicapped' within the community required objective study by concerned, thoughtful and caring people, who understood the problems of individuals who were mentally handicapped, who understood their complex society, who in seeking to enrich the quality of life for the individual also sought to afford them such protection as was possible.

In 1978, following upon discussions with Costello Educational Publishers, the opportunity arose to produce a series of up-to-date reviews of all significant aspects of work in the area of mental retardation. It was agreed that sex education and counselling were amongst the most relevant and urgent of themes. In undertaking this review Ann and Michael Craft have here brought together a cluster of contributions from caring and competent colleagues. Whilst the mildly handicapped will be a major area of concern amongst parents and teachers, attitudes towards the sexuality of the more severely handicapped do not escape challenge.

This book is presented to an international readership in the consciousness that professionals have to consider the needs of today's adults as well as those who will live in the more tolerant society of tomorrow. Whilst there is room in our society for many different approaches to sex education; whilst there will be disagreement with some of the views or suggestions implicit in some of the contributions to this publication; this book will be read with profit by those who wish to face the issue rather than to wish it away. It is a significant contribution to discussion of this area, not an end to it. Its value will be assessed in accordance with the situations, and cultures in which parents and professionals find themselves.

CHAPTER 1

Sexuality and Mental Retardation: a Review of the Literature*

Ann Craft

Introduction

Many sources tell us that we are in the middle of a sexual revolution, a revolution which has changed our attitudes and our behaviour. Debate rages as to the health and wisdom of such change (Gebhard 1980). Certainly, there has been a major shift of emphasis concerning the sexuality of mentally handicapped people. Whereas the early literature concentrated mainly on the *negative* consequences of sexual activity of those deemed mentally defective (significantly joining them to the catgory of morally defective), later authors, write mainly in the context of the *positive* results of aiding mentally handicapped people to live sexually satisfying lives. The early literature may be said to be orientated towards the community standpoint—"the good of society" being the primary consideration. More currently, the philosophical approach is the normalization of life in all its aspects, the rights of mentally handicapped people as individual human beings. Of course the two approaches are not mutually incompatible, although it has sometimes seemed like it.

Kempton (1976) points out that many categories of people have been, or still are, socially oppressed, and vilified or deprived in their attempts to express their sexuality, but she goes on to say that "no group of individuals have been more drastically oppressed because of the *mere fact that they are sexual* than those who are labeled 'retarded'." The Eugenics movement in the first decades of this century had the support of many leading thinkers and intellectuals who feared that "the propagation of the unfit" would swamp society with less able citizens (MacKenzie and MacKenzie 1977).

---

*An abridged version of this review appeared in *Brit. J. Psychiat.* (1981) *139, 494–505*.

1

It was the obvious link between sexual activity and procreation which lent strength to the argument, coupled with an imperfect understanding of the laws of genetic inheritance. Although this understanding is still by no means complete, we do now know that due to random genetic factors, the majority of severely mentally and physically handicapped children are born to normal parents, and we also now have available a range of effective contraceptive methods. Sexual activity need no longer result in pregnancy, and the pregnancy of a handicapped woman does not necessarily mean the birth of a handicapped child.

Better understanding as to how mental handicap arises has played a part in the growth of the normalization philosophy, although of course the philosophy arose from a whole movement towards individual liberty. Many have spelled out what normalization means with regard to the sexuality of mentally handicapped people, and the main points are worth listing:

(1) The right to receive training in social-sexual behaviour that will open more doors for social contact with people in the community.
(2) The right to all the knowledge about sexuality they can comprehend.
(3) The right to enjoy love and to be loved by the opposite sex, including sexual fulfilment.
(4) The right for the opportunity to express sexual impulses in the same form that are socially acceptable for others.
(5) The right to birth control services which are specialized to meet their needs.
(6) The right to marry.
(7) The right to have a voice in whether or not they should have children.
(8) The right for supportive services which involve those rights as they are needed and feasible. (Kempton 1977a; UN 1971.)

We can see how such rights satisfy both "the good of society" and individual freedom, for with teaching, training and the availability of specific support services, the individual is far less likely to clash with the community at large. Nothing, however, is clear cut. Much of the literature reflects a mingling of the old fears and anxieties with a desire to channel positively the sexuality which is inherent in every human, 'handicapped' or 'normal'.

Society's Attitude to the Sexuality of Mentally Handicapped People

Traditionally the sexuality of mentally handicapped people was feared by those who made the rules governing western societies. Where sexual needs were admitted at all, rigid strictures were laid down in order to prevent the mentally handicapped members of a society from procreating. Thus arose the segregated and isolated colonies for defectives, prohibitions on marriages (Berg and Nyland 1973; Grunewald and Linner 1979) and laws permitting sterilization of the mentally incompetent which became widespread, particularly in the USA. The reasons for sterilization were summed up in the much quoted judgement of Justice Oliver Wendell Holmes:

> It is better for all the world, if, instead of waiting to execute degenerate offspring for crimes, or to let them starve for their imbecility, society can prevent those who are manifestly unfit from continuing their kind. The principle that sustains compulsory vaccination is broad enough to cover cutting the fallopian tubes . . . three generations of imbeciles are enough. (*Buck v Bell,* 274 US 200 (1927).)

Sterilizations continued, even though evidence to demonstrate their effectiveness in preventing the birth of mentally handicapped children was lacking (Grunwald 1979). In 1973 Cooke reported that in America:

> Surgical sterilization for the mentally retarded is permitted by statute in 28 states. In 23 of these states, it can be performed without consent. Even when permission is required, institutions frequently utilize coercive measures, such as offering discharge from the institution or the opportunity for marriage, greater freedom and the like, in exchange for agreement to be sterilized.

The issue requires legal clarification as a number of conflicting judgements have been given in American courts (Bayles 1978). The issue is no less cloudy in Britain, where many professionals are uncertain as to the wisest course to pursue (see section on sterilization below, and chapter 11).

Mention has been made of the mentally handicapped as a sexually oppressed group (Kempton 1976). As Hall (1975) points out "behavior which is acceptable when practised by a normal person sometimes becomes unacceptable when practised by someone who is different." Although the 'normal' socio-sexual model is to find a mate, marry and have children, when a retarded person expresses, or worse, acts out these desires, many people perceive it as excessive or shocking (Goodman 1975; Hall 1975).

That a change is coming about in society's attitude to sexual expression by its retarded members, is evident from the volume of literature which aims at enabling mentally handicapped people to develop their potential for loving relationships in ways which are socially acceptable (see for example Lee and Katz 1974).

Parental Attitudes

It would be unfair to look at the attitudes of parents towards the sexuality of their mentally handicapped offspring in isolation, for we know from many sources (media, novels, autobiographies) that parents generally are not good at helping their children achieve physo-sexual maturity. Many a child gets there *in spite of* rather than *because of* parents. While there are good intentions to answer questions honestly, to "have a good talk" man to man or woman to woman, somehow the time is never right. Farrell (1978) reported that while a majority of parents feel they ought to be involved in telling their children about reproduction and sex, only a minority had actually done so.

However, while parents of normal parents usually approve of sex education having a place in secondary schools (Farrell 1978) some parents of retarded children may hold such deep feelings about the sexuality of their child, that they oppose such programmes (Dupras and Tremblay 1976). One of the reasons for this is because, as Pauline Fairbrother amplifies later in this book (chapter 5), many parents of mentally handicapped individuals believe they are lifelong children, with all the innocence that implies. As one parent wrote "If they are innocent, let them stay that way. We hope no over-zealous leader or teacher will try to put any 'big ideas' into a sweet, child-like mind." (Alcorn 1974.) This may not be the majority view, but we do know that parents of retarded children often have particular difficulties in coping with physical and emotional development. As Hammar *et al* (1967) comment, "Puberty and the process of sexual maturation of the retardate created a stressful situation which most families were ill prepared to handle." Watson and Rogers (1980) found that parents of ESN(M) children predicted sexual life events (eg dating, marriage) far later in life than for normal children.

4

What is certain is that sexuality is a major concern for parents, generally focussing around sexual ignorance (and therefore exploitation) and real or anticipated inappropriate behaviour (Hammar *et al* 1967; Kempton and Forman 1976). There are parents who welcome with relief the initiation of schools in setting up sex education programmes (Kempton 1978). Watson and Rogers (1980) found that 88 per cent of parents of ESN(M) children approved of a school giving sex education, with a particular request for teaching of methods of contraception.

Professional Attitudes

As Hall and Sawyer (1978) point out "Any discussion of sexuality of mentally retarded persons includes the sensitive issues which are daily confronting those who come in contact with the retarded population." Sexuality can present management problems in any residential system, be it boarding school or old people's home, but it is a particularly sensitive area where retarded persons are concerned. Mentally handicapped people in hostels and institutions by definition are seen as needing a degree of care and attention. Staff often feel themselves responsible for all areas of residents' lives, and this is reinforced by the attitude of parents and management committees alike. A very high standard of moral behaviour is the expectation, and as Greengross (1976) reminds us, staff feel themselves under pressure to avoid any hint of scandal which might damage the unit's public reputation. All too easily this can result in a devaluing, if not actual repression of sexuality which automatically means that any such expression is seen in terms of a 'problem' for which a 'solution' must be found, the 'solution' looked for being a cessation of the behaviour. The other side of this particular coin is the tendency for professionals to assume that they have the right to make the sexual behaviour of mentally handicapped people their business, sometimes to the extent of deciding what is best without consulting the retarded person at all (Geraghty 1979).

This touches a wider issue, for in a very real way professionals make difficulties for themselves by overprotecting and overcontrolling mentally handicapped residents and clients. Our care systems tend to produce people who are amenable to discipline and who respond well to authoritative direction. We are not so good at enabling people to become more self-sufficient and to assume more personal responsibility. In general we find it hard as caring professionals to let people make their own mistakes and thus we deny them "the dignity of risk" (Perske 1972).

There have been several surveys of the response of residential staff to the sexual behaviour of mentally handicapped people. Mulhern (1975) found that while 67 per cent of respondents felt that sexual frustration contributed to a significant or major degree to most retarded people's problems of adjustment, the only forms of sexual release that received a majority endorsement were private masturbation, brief kissing in private or public and private petting. Mulhern makes the wry observation that, "A commitment to principles of normalization encounters severe strains in the area of sexual behavior." Mitchell *et al* (1978) administered a multi-dimensional questionnaire to staff in three residential facilities for retarded persons to determine their attitudes towards actual and potential sexual behaviour of residents. It was found that 31.2 per cent felt *no* sexual behaviour, not even simple physical contact, was acceptable. This indicates that sex education programmes are likely to meet with resistance by a substantial percentage of staff. Another American survey conducted by Saunders (1979) seemed to show a high tolerance by staff of residents' sexual behaviour and expressed significant interest in assisting residents to cope responsibly with their sexual feelings and sexual behaviour. In Britain the Report of the Jay Committee (DHSS 1979) found that of staff questioned, one quarter of nurses in institutions and one fifth of hostel staff thought that adult residents should be discouraged from developing sexual relationships. Interviews with staff seemed to suggest that their general worries about the sexual behaviour of mentally handicapped people are linked to specific difficulties within their own units. The Report goes on "This would imply that in the future it may become even more important to ensure that nurses and care staff are given an adequate training on sexual behaviour and ways of counselling the mentally handicapped."

The question of formal policies and guidelines is becoming of increasing importance. As Livock (1979) asks "How can staff begin to help the mentally handicapped achieve a coherent model of personal sexual behaviour without the prerequisite of consistant reaction to the sensitive subject from superiors at all levels in the face of any situations and even the most adverse public comment?"

6

Hall and Sawyer (1978) indicate the scope of such policies:

> Institutional facilities and community programs need to develop guidelines which establish sexual policies for their mentally retarded clients which foster rather than hamper individual development. The establishment of such policies should preclude the unnecessary and unfair intervention of staff or helping personnel in the sexual or familial lives of their retarded clients; such policies need to be explicitly stated and carefully adhered to by those charged with the care and training of retarded clients.

What is the position in practice? Mulhern (1975) found that although 70 per cent of the respondents on his survey would have liked a delineated set of guidelines concerning the sexual behaviour of residents, only 23 per cent of units had such policies. In the survey by Saunders (1979) 63 per cent of respondents reported that their facilities had a policy governing the sexual conduct of residents. However:

> Staff members in each of the four facilities contradicted one another in defining the visitation and sexual behavior policies in their facilities, suggesting that either the administration had not circulated to all staff members standards for resident visitation and sexual conduct, or that staff members ignored the written policies in favour of rules of their own convenience and attitudes.

There are some hopeful developments. Hall and Sawyer (1978) report on a workshop format designed to develop sexual behaviour guidelines, and Hall (1978) gives details of a training workshop designed to increase acceptance of sexual expression by mentally handicapped people. In Britain in recent years there has been an increasing number of conferences and workshops on sexuality and mental handicap run especially for staff (for instance the British Institute of Mental Handicap, The Family Planning Association, Castle Priory). There is also a new awareness that education and counselling on sexual matters should be offered by any mental handicap care system to retarded clients, their parents and care staff (NDG 1980).

Wilson and Baldwin (1976) compared staff from an American state institution for the mentally retarded who volunteered for a training workshop in sexuality with staff who did not. While they found that the volunteers significantly improved their knowledge about human sexuality and modified their attitudes towards its expression, they make the important point that:

> If sexuality training for the staff is voluntary, a self-selection process may result in a disproportionate number of participants with more tolerant attitudes about sexuality than non-participants. One potential effect of voluntary training is a polarization of the staff into factions with differing levels of tolerance toward sexuality that may subsequently interfere with positive institutional change.

Attitude of Mentally Handicapped People Towards Sexual Expression

The one thing that can be said with any certainty is that we really know very little about the attitudes of mentally handicapped people towards sexuality in general and their own sexuality in particular. Whittemore and Koegel (1978) make the very relevant observation that while medical, educational and sociological literature all have something to say about sexuality of mentally handicapped people, there is a consistent and striking absence of the motivations and emotions of mentally retarded individuals. As they say:

> Failure of parents and professionals to heed this key dimension threatens to jeopardize success of intervention programs for the mentally retarded. The settings can be provided, but their usefulness depends on the mentally retarded individuals' personal awareness of sexual expressiveness in a social context.

Watson and Rogers (1980) also note that besides an absence of information about sex education in ESN(M) schools there has been a lack of regard to the attitudes of the children themselves. They devised a research instrument to measure knowledge and attitude. In each of four scales the ESN children were significantly more traditional in their attitudes than the normal control subjects. These conservative attitudes may be encouraged by staff and parents as a form of protection, but there may be a potentially dangerousness disjunction between the child and the world outside. They suggest that these mildly retarded youngsters "have the kinds of levels of sexual awareness which were typical of normal adolescents about two decades ago." But whereas for the normal young person in the 1950s there was a degree of match between the prevailing social atmosphere and his own sexual conscience, in the 1980s the world has moved on, norms have changed and the handicapped youngster is far more likely to be confused and inadequate in his sociosexual role when the teaching model tends to be "do as I say, not as I do".

8

What literature there is seems to point to a conservatism of opinion and attitude, perhaps not surprising when we consider the generally conservative views of significant adults in the lives of mentally handicapped people. Edgerton and Dingman (1964) noted that residents in a large mental handicap hospital evolved strict, puritanical rules of conduct to govern sexual behaviour and that transgressors felt guilty and were treated as such by fellow residents. Hall *et al* (1973) also noted a tendency for the mildly retarded adolescent to be conservative in sexual attitude.

Mattison had the impression that sexual intercourse was infrequent among the married couples she surveyed, it was the human warmth and cuddling which was of greater importance (de la Cruz and LaVeck 1973). Grunewald (1979) reports that in Sweden two retarded people in an institution may live together, but that "Most people living together in this way do not appear to have sexual intercourse with one another . . . " He goes on to say that ". . . many have deeply rooted prejudices about the way babies are conceived and are fearful of sexual contact. Many believe that sexual intercourse is forbidden."

Sexual Development

Studies of sexual maturation show a delay in physical sexual development as IQ decreases, although the various syndromes of mental handicap (except for Down's syndrome) do not seem to account for dissimilar patterns of growth between individuals (Mosier *et al* 1962; Salerno *et al* 1975). Profoundly and severely handicapped people are more likely to be delayed in achieving sexual maturity (Alcorn 1974; Hall 1975) and have less pronounced sexual interest and impulses (Wolfensberger 1972).

The majority of mentally handicapped people are in the mild and moderate range, and most of these develop normal reproductive capacities (Salerno *et al* 1975). As individuals with Down's syndrome make up about one third of the severely retarded population, it is important to note that while there is no reported instance of a Down's syndrome male fathering a child (although erection and ejaculation are possible), most of the females are known to be fertile, and have a 50 per cent risk of producing an infant with the same chromosomal abnormality (Tricomi *et al* 1964; Salerno *et al* 1975). Among syndromes contributing to mental

9

handicap, it is said that the brain damaged female has an earlier menarche than the normal (Dalton and Dalton 1978).

Sexual Behaviour

Environment: Like any other behaviour, sexual responses are learned, shaped and reinforced by environments. Rosen (1975) sum it up thus:

> Sexual behaviors in the handicapped can best be understood, *not* as a diluted approximation of normal psycho sexual adjustment in younger children, but as purposive behaviors learned according to unique experience of the retarded person and the specific environmental influences to which he has been subjected. These include the extremely unnatural stimuli available to him in institutional settings, as well as the motivational and emotional consequences of inadequate learning and family experience in the community. Thus, sexual behavior of the handicapped occur logically as an accommodation to the unique cultural and environmental norms of institutions, trainable classes and sheltered workshops. Viewed from this perspective, the sexual adjustment of mentally handicapped persons is at least as normal for their environment as is the sexual adjustment of non-handicapped populations in a more natural environment.

The mentally handicapped see films, watch television series about family situations, look at advertisements, but while many of their expectations may be formed by these influences, the opportunity to fulfil them in socially acceptable ways and settings is often lacking (Sandtner 1972). Institutions may not be good at training people as to what constitutes acceptable and unacceptable sexual behaviour. For instance sex related behaviour such as indiscriminate or inappropriate displays of affection, or open masturbation, may be tolerated, whereas in a community setting, it may not be just embarrassing, but dangerous or illegal (Rosen 1975).

Lack of privacy in the living situation can mean that sexual behaviour is inevitably visible and public. That is not to say that such behaviour does not then constitute a genuine problem, but it does remind us that we have to look carefully at the environment in which behaviour takes place. We also need to look at what precedes and what follows 'problem' sexual behaviour. An excellent manual has been devised for this purpose by Mitchell *et al.* (undated).

Improving Behaviour: Inappropriate sexual conduct may be eliminated by various behaviour therapy techniques, with the

10

substitution or reinforcement of appropriate behaviour. For instance, Polvinale and Lutzker (1980) report success in eliminating the inappropriate interpersonal sexual behaviour and genital self-stimulation of a thirteen year old Down's syndrome boy at school. Foxx (1976) successfully eliminated the public disrobing of a group of mentally handicapped women, and Rosen (1970) describes a technique to condition more appropriate heterosexual behaviour (see also chapter 9). For a discussion of ethical considerations see p 208.

Such techniques, together with the wide-ranging sex education programmes which should accompany them, can go a long way to help the mentally handicapped in two important aspects of sexual behaviour that we have yet to consider—the retarded person as the victim of sexual exploitation and crime, and the retarded person as the sexual offender.

Sexual exploitation: People who are poorly acquainted with the sexual rules of the society in which they live are likely to become victims of sexual exploitation (Kempton 1977a). Mentally handicapped individuals tend to be non-assertive and to agree to participate in sexual acts if directed to do so, possessing poor judgement in assessing other people's motives. There is some evidence that a mentally handicapped person is an ideal victim, for their complaints are not always taken seriously (Kempton and Forman 1976).

Sexual offences: The early view was unequivocal:

> . . . there is no investigator who denies the fearful role played by mental deficiency in the production of vice, crime and delinquency . . . Not all criminals are feeble-minded, but all feeble-minded are at least potential criminals. That every feeble-minded woman is a potential prostitute would hardly be disputed by anyone. (Terman 1916)

When Alfred Binet first developed his original IQ test it was to distinguish between illiterate criminals labelled mentally defective—many for sexual crimes—and others. Even now, depending on the social and IQ variables used, the proportion of convicted offenders found to be defective can range from 2.6 per cent to 39.6 per cent from one American state to another (MacEachron 1979). This researcher found that when IQ testing of all convicts was done the prevalence rate of mentally retarded adult male offenders under IQ 70 is only slightly higher than the prevalence rate of retarded male adults in the general population. She concludes "Social and legal variables are more germane to the problem of being an offender than is intelligence."

No study to date has satisfactorily explored the subject of sexual offences committed by mentally handicapped persons. Brown and Courtless (1968), looking at jailed offenders under IQ 55, did not separate out sexual offences from other crimes against the person, such as homicide and assault. They make the general observation that offences of a sexual nature were the least frequently committed crime by incarcerated offenders under IQ 70. Meyerowitz (1971) claims that almost a third of the charges lodged against the retarded are sexually related, but gives no basis for his figures. Walker and McCabe (1973) using MHA 1959 classifications found that males labelled subnormal and severely subnormal made up one-third of their sample of offenders, but accounted for 50 per cent of the sexual offences. This may seem a clear enough indication, but Parker (1974) in her survey of Special Hospital patients, found 69 per cent of those with a MHA classification of SSN had IQs above 50, which is the normally accepted cut-off IQ point. Of this 69 per cent 3 per cent had IQs above 80. Of those patients with a MHA classification of SN 51 per cent had scores above the normally accepted cut-off point of IQ 70. As Fowles (1977) points out, the classification *subnormal* is commonly interchangeable with *psychopath* in court practice and bears little relation to intellectual retardation, so that all British analyses of offences committed by "subnormals" should be regarded with suspicion in the absence of an IQ rating which would confirm mental handicap.

Two other germane points concern police action. It is often easy to persuade the handicapped to a confession of doubtful veracity, only recently have confessions by a mildly mentally handicapped person without a guardian or professional present, been questioned by British courts. Secondly, motivation: when is an offence a perversion or done with malicious intent, and when it is a result of ignorance and lack of training? As Kempton (1977b) notes, many 'crimes' look much worse on paper than they are in fact. For example, a charge of indecent exposure may result from a retarded man not knowing how to locate a toilet when he is out and urinating in the street. It is impossible to tease out from criminal statistics those 'indecent exposures' from men who deliberately expose themselves for the thrill they get from the reaction of others; or from a retarded adolescent who used an antisocial behaviour which happens to be sexual to get his neighbourhood to notice him. All give cause for concern, but require a different response from parents and professionals (Craft and Craft, 1979a).

Knowledge About Sex

Kempton (1972) has noted some of the reasons why mentally handicapped people tend to have only partial and inaccurate knowledge about sexuality. They are often treated as perpetual children, who should have no interest in sexual matters; their peers (a source of information for normal youngsters) are likely to be equally ignorant; and they usually lack the degree of literacy necessary to find out for themselves from written sources. Edmonson and Wish (1975) looked at 18 institutionalized men aged between 18 and 30 years and commented:

> Serious errors of fact and conceptual confusion, though most prevalent in responses by the low comprehenders, were found in at least some responses by all the men.

and also:

> Like young children, who have not yet acquired a cognitive program of probabilities, they seem untroubled by partial interpretations that are inconsistent with one another, but are highly improbable or impossible.

In the survey by Watson and Rogers (1980) the ESN(M) pupils had significantly less knowledge about sex than the normal control group. Hall and Morris (1976) compared two groups of mentally retarded adolescents, half of whom lived in institutions, and half who were non-institutionalized. The results show that those in institutions showed considerably less knowledge on socio-sexual topics than the mentally retarded living at home. Significantly, the amount of knowledge appeared to decrease with increasing time spent in the residential units, and this in spite of the fact that the units had family life/sex education programmes. The at-home adolescents had far more knowledge about sex roles and family dynamics. Fischer and Krajicek (1974) found that parents were often surprised at the amount of knowledge that their children possessed, but point out that "much depends on the adults' willingness to 'give the child permission' to ask questions or to simply 'wonder' about something of a sexually related nature."

They also make the important point that children generally used colloquial terminology and did not recognize words such as 'masturbation' or 'urination'.

Edmonson *et al* (1979) noted that differences in knowledge were related to the sex of the respondents, their place of residence (institution or community), and past experiences and instruction, rather than to intellectual level. They used the Socio-Sexual Knowledge and Attitudes Test which has been specially developed for developmentally disabled subjects (Wish *et al* 1980) and found that overall the respondents were least well informed about birth control and venereal disease.

Brown's (1980) survey of 16 year old mentally and physically handicapped spastics revealed that while most had a vague but substantially correct idea about the mother's role in pregnancy and birth, only 1 boy out of 31 knew something about menstruation, and only 9 boys knew of the father's role in conception. (See also chapter 7.)

Kempton (1976) reports that it is not unusual to find retarded couples who do not know that sexual intercourse exists. There are also retarded women who believe all sexual intercourse is intended to hurt the female, and have therefore endured all kinds of unpleasant sexual experiences. Sexual ignorance can be a personally impoverishing condition. It can also be dangerous and facilitate exploitation. Very rarely is it a blessing.

For instruments to ascertain the knowledge and attitudes of mentally handicapped people towards sexuality, see Fischer *et al* (1974); Wish *et al* (1980); and Watson and Rogers (1980).

Sex Education

What is Sex Education?

Harris (1974); Reich and Harshman (1971); and Shindell (1975) discuss the goals and objectives of any sex education and are in general agreement that such education should aim at the development of sexually fulfilled persons who understand themselves, their values and resulting behaviours. Kempton (1977b) suggests that the term *sex education* is in fact too limiting for the practical tasks of improving the social-sexual functioning of retarded adolescents. Training in many basic social skills which are only loosely related to sexuality, is needed, and she believes a term such as *socialization education* more nearly encompasses the needs of mentally handicapped people. This view is confirmed by the responses of teachers, surveyed by Watson (1980).

Most authors are agreed that sex education should not be confined to crisis responses to a sexual 'problem,' nor to negative teaching which seeks to prevent any sexual experiences (Edmonson and Wish 1975; Craft and Craft 1978, 1980).

Why do Mentally Handicapped People need Sex Education?

The reasons for, and purpose of, sex education for mentally handicapped people have been well discussed (see Kempton and Forman 1976; Craft and Craft 1978; Johnson 1973; Gordon 1972, 1975). The main points are that the vast majority of retarded people will develop normal secondary sexual characteristics and they need more help not less in understanding these changes and the accompanying emotions. They need knowledge which will give them some protection against exploitation. And lastly, it is unrealistic of society to demand responsible sexual behaviour from people who have never been taught what constitutes responsibility and irresponsibility in sexual matters.

General Position of Sex Education

Until comparatively recently sex education of normal children was haphazard and generally unsatisfactory. Schofield's (1968) survey of young people showed that too little had come too late. Nor is the current position a model of perfection. A report commissioned by the World Health Organization (Isaev, 1979) commented on the paucity of provision in several European countries; Farrell's (1978) report showed that little progress had been made in Britain, and Gebhard (1980) reveals the narrowness of subjects covered in some American states.

Watson and Rogers (1980) surveyed 231 ESN(M) secondary schools in Britain, looking at their sex education programmes, and comparing educational approaches, parental expectations and pupil knowledge and attitude. They could classify the different schools according to the approaches they had adopted to the subject. Those using the *moral* approach relied on the 'inertia' of the ESN(M) adolescent, and would advise strongly against, for instance, premarital sexual intercourse. Because the emphasis was on 'don't'

15

there was a negative corollation with information about contraception and sexually transmitted diseases. The schools using the *relationship approach* emphasised family life, relationships and parenthood, but in rather vague terms, stopping short of specific instruction on contraception, reproduction and sexually transmitted diseases. The third category adopted the *forthcoming approach,* scheduling topics such as relations, contraception, premarital sex and raising issues such as homosexuality and abortion if the students did not. Grunewald and Linner (1979) report that in Sweden sex education is provided to all handicapped students on the same terms as it is to other children of comparable age. It is recognised that many handicapped students will need individual counselling and sometimes expert advice.

Curricula and Resources

Over recent years curricula specially designed for mentally handicapped students have appeared (Craft and Craft 1978; Bender *et al* 1976; Special Education Curriculum Development Centre 1972), together with guides for teachers (Fischer *et al* 1974; Kempton 1975; Kempton and Forman 1976).

Teachers still complain a lack of teaching materials and often resort to making their own, but for a review of helpful audiovisual material available in Britain (see Craft 1980).

Who Teaches?

Watson and Rogers (1980) report that in 31 per cent of the ESN(M) schools surveyed *all* staff were involved in sex education, but that there was usually an understanding that no teacher need take part if they did not wish to do so.

The training and preparation of teachers is obviously a vitally important area. Meyen (1970) and Meyen and Retish (1971) discuss the usefulness of workshops to help teachers realise firstly the need for giving retarded people sex education, then to pick out relevant subject matter, view resource material and perhaps most importantly, discuss and explore personal worries and concerns about such teaching.

Is much being done at the earlier stage of general teacher training? Evidence from one American survey indicated that while 61 per cent of student teachers on special education courses

16

received some preparation in sex education, this preparation was either an elective option or a few hours of coverage fitted in under a different topic, such as methods of teaching. It is probable that the position in Britain is similar. May (1980) suggests several ways in which facilities responsible for the training of special school teachers could offer better coverage of this vital area.

In locations other than schools the profession of the person who undertakes the teaching is of minor importance. The essential point is that the person concerned is at ease with the subject and the students, and has the approval of the managing authority (Craft and Craft, 1978; Kempton, 1972).

What Effect does Teaching Have?

One worry that many teachers share with parents is that giving the mentally handicapped youngster sex education will trigger sexual experimentation and appetite, opening up a Pandora's box that should have been kept tightly closed. On the contrary, two of the foremost American experts in the field claim that the opposite occurs. In the words of Sol Gordon (1975) "Information inhibits behavior; knowledge causes people to be a little bit more introspective; it makes them think." Winifred Kempton (1978) in an evaluation of 31 courses that showed her slides on *Sexuality and the Mentally Handicapped* to a total of 430 retarded students said that, "There were no reports that the staff was aware of serious inappropriate behavior that could be attributed to the programs." What teachers did report was an improvement in social behaviour, increase self-respect, more openness, and fewer feelings of guilt.

The argument of letting sleeping dogs lie has a false premise anyway because it implies that 'not telling' means 'no one does anything'. This simply is not so, for there is plenty of evidence that withholding information does not deter sexual activity (Kempton and Forman, 1976). Rather it causes confusion, needless fears, inappropriate behaviour and unwanted consequences (sometimes as serious as pregnancy).

We need to be realistic in our expectations of the effect of sex education. Environments are powerful shapers of behaviour. As one of the teachers on Watson's (1980) survey commented, "The majority of our pupils will behave in accordance with the mores of their social group." There was evidence to show that teachers were

17

significant in aiding 'survival'—half the ESN(M) students said it was 'teacher' who had taught them about sex. This group scored significantly higher on the knowledge scale than those taught by 'family or friend' and were less punative in their attitudes towards masturbation and sexuality. In particular, leavers who had been given sex education showed less anxiety than those who had not.

The Effect of Handicap on Learning

We know from educational research that retarded students have particular difficulties in learning (Mittler 1979) characterized as they are by poor cognitive skills and limited attention spans. In addition they are likely to have secondary handicaps of a sensory or physical nature. All combine to make teaching a complex task. In the context of sex education Watson and Rogers (1980) comment, "The problem here is that while skilled teaching may enable *specific ability* to be achieved in such areas as contraceptive use or awareness of sexually transmitted diseases, it can do little to raise the *levels of reasoning.*" However, as they go on to point out, ". . . until sexual instruction for these young people has been fully developed as an educational technology (from teacher training to the availability of suitable teaching aids) the limits of achievement will not be known."

The Parents' Part in Sex Education

As we have seen in the section on parental attitudes, this is an area that many parents find particularly stressful, whether their children are handicapped or not. Several books have been written specifically for parents of mentally handicapped children, and among the most helpful are Kempton *et al* (1972); Gordon (1973); Lee (1976); and Shennan (1976).

Of the parents of the ESN(M) childrn on the Watson and Roger's (1980) survey, 88 per cent wanted their offspring to have sex education at school, or home and school together, and 43 per cent stated that they found it hard to talk about sex to their children. Not surprisingly, the parents were most keen to have the children taught about contraception.

Sex Education of Severely Mentally Handicapped People

Most of the foregoing discussion has primarily concerned those who are mildly or moderately retarded. They are, after all, in the numerical majority of the handicapped population. The profoundly and severely mentally handicapped are sometimes in danger of having their needs passed over. There may well be different priorities, but they too have sexual needs and require a form of sex education. This education is more in the nature of training in areas such as proper hygiene, proper techniques and places for masturbation, and socially acceptable methods of physical contact with others (Kempton 1977b). Spontaneous sexual activities are almost entirely confined to auto-eroticism.

Hamre-Nietupski and Williams (1977) and Hamre-Nietupski and Ford (1981) describe in helpful detail the successful implementation of a programme for severely handicapped students incorporating basic sex education and social skills with self-care, language and home living skills. Good co-operation between parents and teachers was achieved. The teacher's manual by Bender *et al* (1976) contains graded programmes for teaching social skills, body functions, etc., and that devised by the Special Education Curriculum Development Centre (1972) has suggestions of teaching objectives and methods which might be employed with severely retarded students. In Britain the Inner London Education Authority currently has a working party looking at the whole question of health and sex education for ESN(S) pupils. Besides guidelines for schools, it is hoped that the group will produce some teaching material.

Conclusion

The status of the sex education of retarded students and the dilemma currently (perhaps habitually) facing those who undertake the task have been well summed up by Watson and Rogers (1980):

> The uniquely difficult task facing the sex educator of the ESN(M) is how to develop sufficient knowledge and a solid enough attitudinal basis to enable such a group of break away from adult dependence, to experience normal adolescent rebellion, to experiment with socio-sexual relationships (in short to be as normal as possible) without becoming sexual casualties. Our data suggests that there is still a very long way to go before such a goal is reached.

Marriage

As previously mentioned, it was the association of marriage with parenthood that prompted the Eugenicists' argument and led to laws on sterilization and on the prohibition of marriages in an effort to reduce the frequency of handicap in the population. In Denmark the law until recently forbade all mentally handicapped persons to marry, unless they had special permission from the Ministry of Justice (Bank-Mikkelsen 1973). Restrictions were also imposed in Sweden (Grunewald and Linner 1979). Now improved methods of birth control are available to everyone, and no one need produce children they do not want, or more children than they can cope with. Yet still society tends to impose a double standard on mentally handicapped citizens. As Wolfensberger (1972) comments:

> There are many nonretarded, physically healthy people who are sex driven, shallow, incompetent, unstable and incapable of deep, even of sustained relationships, yet our political system accords them the constitutional right to enter a legal marriage. In our society, a citizen has the right to treat sex on the 'itch-and-scratch' level, and to enter a legal marriage that does not rise above this level. Therefore, we should either apply more stringent criteria to *all* citizens, or cease applying them to the handicapped . . . if it [marriage] is an act available to citizens who are not impaired, it should also be available to those who are impaired.

The literature concerning marriages where both partners have been labelled mentally handicapped does not necessarily distinguish between those under IQ 70 and those hospitalized with personality disorders, who often reached average ability (IQ 90-100) after a turbulent adolescence. Mattinson (1975) followed up discharged hospital residents known to have married other ex-mental handicap hospital patients. Of the 80 original subjects, 16 had IQs of over 70, 21 had IQs between 60 and 69 with scores likely to have been depressed by upbringing and the anxiety engendered by the admission. Floor *et al* (1975) surveyed 214 discharges from an American institution, 80 of whom had married. The mean IQ on discharge was 76 (male 78.1; female 71.3).

As with Mattinson's group, they were mostly people with no family, or uninterested families, admitted because they were social nuisances. Berry and Shapiro (1975) looked at 19 marriages where both partners had been in mental handicap hospitals. The average IQ was 69 (male 74; female 63). In Shaw and Wright's (1960) Sheffield study 11 per cent of their sample had IQs above 69. Craft and Craft (1979b) followed up 45 marriages where one or both partners had IQs below 70.

Is it possible to predict whether a marriage involving mentally hanicapped people will succeed? In fact there are methodological difficulties in any prediction of social adaptation (for a discussion see Edgerton and Bercovici 1976). In a survey of patients discharged from a mental handicap hospital, Edgerton (1967) noted:

> It would seem that the sexual and marital lives of these retarded persons are more 'normal' and better regulated than we could possibly have predicted from the knowledge of their pre-hospital experiences and their manifest intellectual deficits.

Mattinson (1975) looked at four obvious factors which might have a predictive value—recorded IQ, length of time spent in hospital, behaviour in hospital, and early history and background of deprivation. None of these factors correlated significantly with the achievement scores obtained by the 32 couples on her survey. Berg and Nyland (1973) say of their Danish couples, "that a common life has had a positive or stabilizing effect on social deviations." Hall (1974) lists 18 factors appearing in the literature, which if present in significant numbers and/or degrees can effect the 'success' of the marriage involving a retarded individual. Among these are emotional disturbance of one or both partners; faulty childhood background; both partners being retarded; and length of institutionalization. As might be expected, many of these 18 factors have a bearing on the stability of any marriage, but the reactions of human beings to each other and to circumstances are often *not* predictable. In one of the marriages surveyed by Craft and Craft (1979b) nine of these adverse factors were present. Both the mentally handicapped wife and her schizophrenic husband acknowledged the partnership to be unsatisfactory, but they had resolutely clung to each other for the 27 years of their marriage. As Hall (1974) says, "Certain needs may be met in a marital partnership that cannot be met elsewhere."

Several studies have stressed the importance of the support a couple receives in day-to-day living. This may be from an official agency or a private person, someone Edgerton (1967) calls a 'befriender'. All but one of the 12 couples on Andron and Sturm's (1973) survey depended upon other people in varying degrees for everything from advice to money. Of the Danish couples, two thirds looked after their homes without any help, but just over a third needed help in managing their money (Berg and Nyland 1973).

Only eight of the 32 couples surveyed by Mattinson (1975) were unknown to any welfare agency. Craft and Craft (1979b) found that 12 of their couples managed everything for themselves, 21 more lived in the community and needed some measure of support from family, friends or professionals.

In the last resort marriage is a contract between two people, and it is the partners themselves who must be the final judges of success or failure. Edgerton (1967) reports that marriage for the discharged mentally handicapped person is a highly meaningful status to achieve, it emphasizes a newly won position as a free and full member of the outside world. It is seen as proof of normality. Among Mattinson's (1975) 32 marriages, 25 were considered by the spouses to be preferable to being single. Andron and Sturm (1973) report, "All but one man said that married life was better than single life. The overwhelming reason was the companionship that marriage provided in contrast to their previous social isolation." Craft and Craft (1979b) found that the partners in 35 of the 41 intact marriages preferred their present status to their single existance. As one husband put it, "Marriage? It do beat being single!" The reason for this satisfaction, often despite poor material circumstances, is best summed up by Mattinson (1975):

> [the] reality was usually so much better than anything they had known before; and an awareness of their limitations and often considerable ignorance of what went on in other people's homes enabled them not to over-reach themselves and search for the finer subtleties of living.

Pre-marital counselling: a pre-marital counselling service for mentally handicapped engaged couples has been described by Craft and Craft (1979a) and also Hartman and Hynes (1975). See also chapter 12 in this book.

Parenthood

The literature explores three aspects—the likelihood that the children of mentally handicapped parents will be retarded themselves; the child rearing abilities of mentally handicapped parents; and fertility with family size.

Risk of Handicap in Offspring

The studies of mentally handicapped parents estimating the percentage of retarded children vary enormously in their findings.

22

Hall (1974) reviewed 31 studies dating from 1913 to 1965. The percentage of mentally handicapped children produced ranged from 2.5 to 93.2. As Hall makes clear, these estimations vary principally because of differences in definition and criteria in the studies themselves. Brandon (1957) found her south London females had 150 pregnancies before and after certification, 24.7 per cent having miscarried or died before two years old. Of 109 surviving children tested, the mean IQ was 91.3, only four consistently scoring below IQ 65. Of children reared by their natural (defective) mother, their mean IQ was 98.7. However, many of the 73 defective mothers were 'social' defectives, well above IQ 70 on initial testing. Shaw and Wright (1960) assess 377 children from married defectives and found 46 'retarded'. However, of children tested, only three children had scored under 70 in both of two IQ tests "which suggests that few mentally retarded children had been overlooked." Many attended ESN schools, but the assessments are not clear. They note "stable mentally defective mothers can cope with . . . one or two children . . .[with more] they become overwhelmed" and "children found neglected were the offspring of defective parents who themselves had an unsatisfactory upbringing." Scally (1973) uses social quotients rather than IQ to evaluate offspring, and is thus very difficult to compare with others.

The most comprehensive analysis of IQ status of parents and children is provided by a population survey from the Minnesota Institute of Human Genetics, looking at records for 7,778 children (Reed and Reed, 1965). In the 89 instances where both parents had IQs under 70, nearly 40 per cent of the children were also educationally retarded (although the average IQ of the children was 74). Where one parent only had an IQ below 70, 15 per cent of the children were retarded (54 per cent had IQs above 90); and of the 7,035 with neither parent retarded, one per cent were mentally handicapped. Surveying their data, they calculated that for a mentally handicapped person under IQ 70, the expectation for one of their children to also consistently score under IQ 70 was 17.1 per cent. Reed and Anderson (1973) constructed a model which predicted that some 17 per cent of mentally handicapped children in any generation would have been produced by the retarded, the remaining 83 per cent having retardation resulting from abnormal mutations, recessive genes and other chance pre- and post-natal factors, produced by persons of normal IQ. Other more recent studies lack adequate criteria. Mattinson (1975) and Craft and Craft (1979b) did not check the IQ of children produced, only noting current educational status.

Parental Competency

Assessing the competence of mentally handicapped parents is a complex matter. Individuals in different strata of society would give different answers to the question of how we judge the adequacy of any parent. The National Child Development study in Britain found that by the age of seven there are major differences between children of different social classes in health, skills and scholastic attainment (Davie *et al* 1972). Shaw and Wright (1960) report that almost a third of their families with one or more children had been reported to the authorities because of neglect or cruelty. As with all surveys, they found that difficulties increased as families got larger. Of the children born to the couples on Mattinson's (1975) survey, six (from three families) had been committed to the care of the local authority, the remaining 34 were being looked after by their parents. Ten of the 13 families with children under school age were receiving regular or intensive support of health visitors or social workers, but none of the children appeared to be in dire need. Berg and Nyland (1973) report that of the 38 children living with their mentally handicapped parents, 21 were receiving good care, two satisfactory care, 11 acceptable care and two bad care (two not known). Of the 30 children born of the marriages Craft and Craft (1979b) followed up, four (of two marriages) were in local authority care, and two children of one family were on the Social Services 'At Risk' register, although still living at home. In all but two of the families with children under the age of twelve, a social worker and/or health visitor gave active support.

We know that physical and emotional environment can play an important part in the development of retardation of intelligence. Much depends on the childhood emotional experience of the mother, and unfortunately many retarded people have had damaging upbringings which make it difficult for them to appreciate their children's needs (Grunewald 1979). In Sweden a vigorous attempt is made to incorporate mentally handicapped mothers into a network of social contacts and to admit the children to day nurseries/kindergartens at an early age. Grunewald (1979) goes on to describe the comprehensive service available to retarded parents (see also Grunewald and Linner 1979). Craft and Craft (1979b) give a detailed case history showing some of the issues involved in supporting mentally handicapped parents.

On the subject of competence Wolfensbergr (1972) makes the apposite comment:

> If unfitness for parenthood becomes a criterion, then it should be applied both to the retarded and nonretarded alike—and many bright, well-educated persons are unfit parents.

With modern positive approaches, how far can the children of mentally handicapped parents be helped in their development? It is generally accepted that at least three-quarters of identified mentally handicapped people under IQ 70 come from the 'cultural-familial' or 'socially deprived' group, having no known organic explanation for their handicap (see Craft 1979). Garber and Heber (1977) report a project to detect those at risk of developing retardation because of their cultural-familial background, and to prevent it happening. The research centred on a Milwaukee slum. The group of children at risk of developing mental retardation was identified with the intention of intervening in their lives prior to the decline in intellectual levels which was detectable from the age of two. Early results are encouraging. At the age of 66 months, the experimental group had a mean score on the Wechsler Preschool and Primary Scale Index of 123 (standard deviation 7.6), while the controls had a mean of 92 (standard deviation 9.4). At 96 months there was a differential of 20 or more points between the two groups. One-third of the controls had IQs below 75 (Wechsler Intelligence Scale for Children); by contrast the lowest IQ scores for the experimental children were two with 88. It remains to be seen whether this ability will be maintained in spite of the continuing adverse social conditions of these children. There was one unexpected development—the experimental children were reported to be having behavioural problems at school. Garber and Heber comment:

> These are usually the result of their high level of verbal behavior, which sharply contrasts with their peers and gives them the ability to confront the teacher. Above all, the Milwaukee Project children were given confidence, skill and practice in the use of language as an effective tool for interacting with the adults in their lives.

The teachers may have put it differently!

Fertility and Family Size

Fertility has two aspects: the biological capacity to reproduce, and effective reproduction (ie the numbers of children actually produced). With regard to the former, most mentally handicapped adults are fertile at a biological level, although there are obvious exceptions such as Klinefelter's and Turner's syndromes. However, the more severe the physical damage, the less is the likelihood of a functioning reproductive system (Wolfensberger 1972). The second aspect becomes a function of drive, opportunity, contraception, or, as in China, politics. In fact a review of the literature over recent years shows family size diminishing faster if anything, among the handicapped than among the general Western population.

In 1959 Wright *el al* could find 319 children, 46 per cent retarded, produced by 61 'defective' couples, whilst Shaw and Wright (1960) found 177 Sheffield defectives producing 377 children (12 per cent retarded). After 20 years of national contraceptive education and social support the picture has greatly changed. Mattinson (1975) reported an average of 1.5 children among her surveyed couples, a mean family size lower than in the comparable general population (2.1). Craft and Craft (1979b) find their 45 couples (defectiveness now defined as under IQ 70) producing but 30 children, and only two couples not using contraception. Grunewald (1979) reports a Swedish decline in births to this at-risk group.

Birth Control

The modern development of safe, reliable and readily available methods of birth control has made an enormous practical difference to mentally handicapped people, and to the people who counsel them. As we have seen, it was fear of the reproductive capacity of the retarded from which stemmed the social policies segregating the sexes in isolated colonies and institutions, backed up in many instances by laws of accepted medical practice facilitating sterilization. The current literature on the subject is now concerned with three main areas:

(a) a discussion of the merits of various methods of birth control for a mentally handicapped population;

(b) delivery of the family planning services to mentally handicapped clients; and

(c) the question of valid consent.

(a) *Suitable Methods*

Just as with the population at large, there is no one preferred contraceptive technique for mentally handicapped people. Age, medical history, ability, living situation and motivation all need to be fully considered.

The Pill: Use of oral contraceptives where there are no medical contra indications presupposes motivation and/or regular supervision. For many mildly retarded women these conditions pertain, and they use the method successfully (Hall 1975; Kempton and Forman 1976; Kempton 1979). There are drawbacks over and above those for the general population—mentally handicapped females may already be taking other prescribed medication such as anti-convulsant drugs, phenothiazines or anti-depressants. In general polypharmacy is best avoided if another method will serve just as well (MacLean 1979).

Intrauterine device (IUD): Hall (1975) considers that the IUD is best suited for a sexually active woman who lacks supervision and sustained motivation. It is also the method preferred by MacLean (1979). One drawback is that the device can be removed by the woman or her partner. To guard against this one clinic cut the threads very short (Maclean 1979). Another danger is that the dislodgement of the device may not be noticed or understood. Not uncommonly mentally handicapped people feel that their genitals are 'dirty' and they are reluctant or afraid to look closely. Check-ups at smaller time intervals would help ensure the IUD remains in place (Kempton and Forman 1976).

Depo-Provera: Use of this drug, which inhibits ovulation, has now been approved by the Committee on Safety of Medicine in Britain on specialist prescription only. One injection every three months is required, but there are some disadvantages, such as breakthrough bleeding and an unpredictable return of fertility after discontinuation (Kempton 1979). Its main usefulness is as a short-term measure, for example, to protect a woman against pregnancy during an episode of disturbed and promiscuous behaviour; or for a wife in the period immediately following her husband's vasectomy.

Other Non-permanent Measures: In general other methods such as the condom, foam and the diaphram are not considered suitable for

27

mentally handicapped people to employ. Gordon (1975) does think retarded males may be able to master the technique of using a condom if it is explained simply and clearly. Of course, to be most efficacious the female partner should use a spermicidal foam, and this may not always be appreciated by the couple.

Sterilization: Because of its permanent effect, this is linked more than any other issue to the question of valid consent (see (c) below). Generally the consensus would seem to be that while sterilization can be recommended to individuals who, after counselling, decide they do not want any more children, or children at all, other alternatives should always be considered first (Hall 1975). There are a number of points to be considered. Parents who request sterilization are often responding to a fear of potential, rather than actual, irresponsible behaviour. They may well genuinely, but erroneously, believe that sterilization removes not only the reproductive capacity, but all sexual drive and impulse. Kempton (1977b) points out that sterilization is usually too drastic a step to take because it is very difficult to predict what an individual's real potential is. Decisions made on the basis of temporary adolescent behaviour may prove wrong in the light of later maturity. With improved methods of training, teaching and treatment, people can and do develop abilities and skills. In Sweden, no-one under 18 can be sterilized (Grunewald and Linner 1979). There are, of course, cases where sterilization is wholly advisable. For instance MacLean (1979) writes of the case of a mildly handicapped woman who had twice killed her children. She was greatly distressed at the thought of ever becoming pregnant again, but after counselling and sterilization was able to live in a stable and supportive relationship with a man. Craft and Craft (1979b) report that several couples on their survey requested sterilization to relieve them of the worry of potential parenthood.

There is one last point to consider—the *subjective* angle. As we know from studies in the general population, there are those who regret having consented to sterilization. There really is no way this occurrence can be guarded against, except by careful and unrushed counselling beforehand. Many of the mentally handicapped are, however, in a different position, legatees of a system in the not-so-distant past that either linked sterilization to discharge from an institution, or claimed to act in the best interest of the retarded, by carrying out the operations under false pretences. Several authors comment on the bitterness and sad regret felt by people treated in this way (Edgerton 1967; Andron and Sturm 1973; Hall 1975). They felt themselves to be stigmatized and cheated.

Abortion: As with the normal population, abortion is hedged by medico-legal safeguards. It is especially appropriate as an option in the cases of exploitation (Kempton 1977a). Grunewald and Linner (1979) describe the position in Sweden and comment that the Swedish legislature in passing the 1975 law on abortion, stressed the need for extending and improving preventative action in the way of birth control advice and sex education. This of course applies equally well to the retarded as to the normal population.

(b) *Effective Delivery of Service*

It is no use having effective methods of birth control if the at-risk population does not avail itself of them. David *et al.* (1976) carried out a pilot scheme to provide a specialised family planning clinic for mentally retarded clients. Recruitment in the Washington DC clinic was disappointingly low. In spite of wide publicity, advertising, direct contact with 37 target institutions and approaches to professionals working with mentally handicapped, only 47 clients were attracted in a seven month period, 41 of them from one institution. MacLean (1979; see also chapter 11) describes a family planning clinic set up several years ago in a hospital for the mentally handicapped. As might be expected, the majority of clients were the mildly handicapped, turbulent younger age group. It seemed sensible to offer such a service where there is a congregation of potential clients. For those mentally handicapped people in the community, local family planning clinics are increasing their expertise in counselling and treating retarded men and women.

(c) *Valid and Informed Consent*

Advocates of the sexual and civil rights of mentally handicapped people have been much exercised on the matter of 'consent', particularly in the case of sterilization which is the most permanent form of birth control (Hastings Center Report 1978; Evans 1980; Gostin 1980), although of course the 'consent' debate is equally pertinent to the prescription of other methods of contraception. Where people are deficient in their intellectual and reasoning ability, there is always a danger of the agents of society assuming global decision-making rights. Add to this the general non-assertiveness of retarded people and the way they are easily influenced by authority figures, and the danger is magnified. The law, and informed current opinion now challenges this assumption of "it is in their best interest", but the question of the 'validity' of consent is a vexed one. A legally effective (or valid) consent has the following elements:

(1) it is voluntary; (2) information is provided about (a) the procedure and possible consequences and (b) alternative procedures and their possible consequences; and (3) the person is capable of comprehending the information (Bayles 1978).

How are these elements dealt with in sterilization decisions? In Britain there is no set procedure, but the judgement given in the court case of *In re D* (a minor) (1976) 1 All ER 326 reminded medical practitioners of the issues involved, particularly where the mentally handicapped person is a minor, for the best interests of parents/guardian may diverge from those of the child. The judge concluded the operation would not be in the best interests of this eleven year old mildly mentally handicapped girl. The judge rejected the pediatrician's proposition that where there is parental consent, the decision to carry out a sterilization operation on a minor was solely within the doctor's clinical judgment, even when the purpose was non-therapeutic (ie not just for the health of the patient).

In America the legal situation remains in need of clarification. In some states courts have ruled that no mentally incompetent person is capable of consenting to sterilization, yet in others the courts permit the state to order sterilization (Bayles 1978; Gostin 1980). The Planned Parenthood Associations in the various states have been active in providing counselling services to candidates for sterilization.

Following a report in 1978 that 686 sterilization operations have been performed in Ontario hospitals on persons unable to give their own consent, the Ontario legislature imposed a moratorium on the sterilization of minors and mentally incompetent persons, except in cases where the operation was "medically necessary for the protection of the physical health of the patient or outpatient." (Evans 1980.) The moratorium has been indefinitely extended. Evans, the general counsel for the Canadian Medical Protective Association writes:

Clearly, when after giving a very clear consideration to the circumstances of the specific request the doctor concludes that the proposed sterilization can be justified only on nonmedical grounds, as a contraceptive measure or for the convenience of the parent or guardian, he must refuse the request. Secondly, in Ontario and probably in all provinces, a doctor should refuse to perform a sterilization procedure on a mentally retarded child under the age of 16 unless the operation is medically necessary for the protection of the *physical* health of the child.

He goes on:

Predictably, there will be differences of opinion as to what properly constitutes a clear medical necessity. Until there is further judicial pronouncement on the subject or some clear and unequivocal statutory legislation in the area, it is difficult to know where the line might be drawn. In the present climate, even in the case of mentally retarded persons over the age of 16 years, it is suggested that the potential of medicolegal problems increases as the doctor moves from the physical to the nonphysical health of the patient as a basis for the medical necessity of the procedure.

In 1979 the Supreme Court of Prince Edward Island rejected an application for the sterilization of a mentally handicapped woman of 24 on the grounds that no clinical therapeutic reasons for the operation had been established.

In Sweden if a mentally handicapped person still lacks an understanding of the consequences of sterilization after discussion and counselling, the operation may not be performed. The onus falls on the doctor to satisfy himself that the applicant understands the situation. He may request a second opinion from a specialist, such as the psychiatrist. Such cases are said to be rare (Grunewald 1979; Grunewald and Linner 1979).

Conclusion

The literature reflects the impact of the philosophy of normalization. Nothing stands still, and we strive to do our best to improve techniques and services. Many of our existing provisions of care and support are rather like the curate's egg, good only in parts. Lip service to the normalization principles which were embodied in the United Nations Declaration of Rights of the Mentally Handicapped is not enough. Livock (1979) for example asks one of the pertinent questions which will exercise us in the next decade; "Is it moral to give mentally handicapped people information about sexuality in a society whose facilities are going to deny the realistic expression of it?" The literature has raised other issues such as the need to develop educational approaches and materials for the slow learner relating to sociosexual knowledge; the inclusion of strategies for sex education in the training courses of special school teachers; the formulation of officially recognized policies and guidelines covering sexual behaviour in residential facilities, together with appropriate staff training; intervention programmes to foster parenting skills; and crucially, discovering and taking notice of mentally handicapped people's own feelings, needs, strivings, ambitions concerning their sexuality. The chapters which follow in this book are addressed to some of these questions, presenting viewpoints, strategies and possible ways forward.

REFERENCES

Alcorn, D.A. (1974). Parental Views on Sexual Development and Education of the Trainable Mentally Retarded. *J. Special Education 8,* 2, 119–130.

Andron, L. and Sturm, M.L. (1973). Is "I do" in the Repertoire of the Retarded? *Ment. Retardation 11,* 31–4.

Bank-Mikkelson, N.E. (1973). Marriage and Mental Retardation in Denmark: Legal and Moral Aspects. Paper given at third congress of International Association for the Scientific Study of Mental Deficiency, The Hague, September 1973.

Bayles, M. (1978). The Legal Precedents. *Hastings Center Report 8,* 3, 37–41.

Bender, M., Valletutti, P.J. and Bender, R. (1976). *Teaching the Moderately and Severely Handicapped.* Volume II: Communication, Socialization, Safety and Leisure Time Skills. Baltimore and London: University Park Press.

Berg, E. and Nyland, D. (1973). Marriage and Mental Retardation in Denmark: A follow-up of mentally retarded applicants for permission to marry. Paper given at third Congress of International Association for the Scientific Study of Mental Deficiency, The Hague, September 1973.

Berry, J.M. and Shapiro, A. (1975). Married Mentally Handicapped Patients in the Community. *Proc. of the Roy.Soc.Med. 68,* 12, 795–8.

Brandon, M.W.G. (1957). The Intellectual and Social Status of Children of Mental Defectives. *J.Ment.Science 103,* 433, 710.

Brown, B.S. and Courtless, T.F. (1968). The Mentally Retarded Offender. In: Allen R.C., Ferster, E.Z. and Rubin, J.A. (eds) *Readings in Law and Psychiatry* Baltimore: Johns Hopkins University Press.

Brown, H. (1980). Sexual Knowlege and Education of ESN Students in Centers of Further Education. *Sexuality and Disability 3,* 3, 215–20.

Cooke, R.E. (1973). Ethics and Laws on behalf of the Mentally Retarded. In: Haslam, R.H.A. (ed) *The Pediatric Clinics of North America 20,* 1, 259–68.

Craft, A. (1980). *Health, Hygiene and Sex Education for Mentally Handicapped Children, Adolescents and Adults: A review of audio-visual resources.* Health Education Council, 71-75 New Oxford Street, London WC1A 1AH.

Craft, A. and Craft, M. (1979a). Personal Relationships and Partnerships for the Mentally Handicapped. In: Craft, M. (ed) *Tredgold's Mental Retardation,* 12th editn. London: Bailliere Tindall.

Craft, A. and Craft, M. (1979b). *Handicapped Married Couples*. London: Routledge and Kegan Paul.

Craft, A. and Craft, M. (1980). Sexuality and the Mentally Handicapped. In: Simon, G.B. (ed) *Modern Management of Mental Handicap: A Manual of Practice*. Lancaster: MTP Press.

Craft, M. (1979) (ed). *Tredgold's Mental Retardation*, 12th editn. London: Bailliere Tindall. pp 10–15, 361.

Craft, M. and Craft, A. (1978). *Sex and the Mentally Handicapped*. London: Routledge and Kegan Paul.

Dalton, M.E. and Dalton, K. (1978). Menarchial age in the disabled. *Brit.Med.J.2*, 475.

David, H.P., Smith, J.D. and Friedman, E. (1976). Family Planning Services for Persons Handicapped by Mental Retardation. *Am.J.Public Health 66*, 11, 1053–7.

Davie, R., Butler, N.R. and Goldstein, H. (1972). *From Birth to Seven*. London: Longmans.

de la Cruz, F.F. and LaVeck, GD. (eds) (1973). *Human Sexuality and the Mentally Retarded*. New York: Brunner/Mazel; London: Butterworths, p 217.

Department of Health and Social Security (1979). *Report of the Committee of Enquiry into Mental Handicap, Nursing and Care* (Jay Committee). Cmnd 7468. London: HMSO.

Dupras, A. and Tremblay, R. (1976). Path Analysis of Parents' Conservatism toward Sex Education of their Mentally Retarded Children. *Am.J.Ment.Defic. 81*, 2, 162–66.

Edgerton, R.B. (1967). *The Cloak of Competence*. London: Cambridge University Press.

Edgerton, R.B. and Bercovici, S.M. (1976). The Cloak of Competence: Years Later. *Am.J.Ment.Defic. 80*, 5, 485–97.

Edgerton, R.B. and Dingman, H.F. (1964). Good Reasons for Bad Supervision: 'dating' in hospital for the mentally retarded. *Psychiatric Quarterly Supplement 38*, 221–33.

Edmondson, B., McCombs, K. and Wish, J. (1979). What Retarded Adults believe about Sex. *Am.J.Ment.Defic. 84*, 11–18.

Edmondson, B. and Wish, J. (1975). Sex Knowledge and Attitudes of Moderately Retarded Males. *Am.J.Ment.Defic. 80*, 2, 172–9.

Evans, K.G. (1980). Sterilization of the Mentally Retarded—A Review. *Can.Med.Assoc.J. 123*, 1066–70.

Farrell, C. (1978). *My Mother Said . . .* London: Routledge and Kegan Paul.

Fischer, H.L. and Krajicek, M.J. (1974). Sexual Development of the Moderately Retarded Child: How Can the Pediatrician be Helpful? *Clin.Pediatrics 13*, 1, 79–83.

Fischer, H.L., Krajicek, M.J. and Borthick, W.A. (1974). *Sex Education for the Developmentally Disabled: A guide for parents, teachers and professionals* (rev ed). Baltimore: University Park Press.

Floor, L., Baxter, D., Rosen, M. and Zisfein, L. (1975). A Survey of Marriages among previously Institutionalized Retardates. *Ment. Retardation 13*, 33–7.

Fowles, M.W. (1977). Sexual Offenders in Rampton. In: Gunn J. (ed) *Sex Offenders —a Symposium*. Special Hospitals Research Report No 14. Special Hospitals Research Unit.

Foxx, R.M. (1976). The Use of Over Correction to Eliminate the Public Disrobing (stripping) of Retarded Women. *Behavior Research and Therapy 14*, 53–61.

Garber, H. and Heber, F.R. (1977). The Milwaukee Project: indications of the effectiveness of early intervention in preventing mental retardation. In: Mittler, P. (ed) *Research to Practice in Mental Retardation*, Vol. I. Baltimore: University Park Press.

Gebhard, P.H. (1980). Sexuality in the Post-Kinsey Era. In: Armytage, W.H.G., Chester, R. and Peel, J. (eds) *Changing Patterns of Sexual Behaviour*. London: Academic Press.

Geraghty, P. (1979). The Joy of Love. *Community Care,* 5 April, 24–5.

Goodman, L. (1972). The Sexual Rights for the Retarded—a dilemma for parents. In: Bass, M.S. and Gelof, M. (eds) *Sexual Rights and Responsibilities of the Mentally Retarded.* Proceedings of the Conference of American Association on Mental Deficiency, Region IX, 1972.

Gordon, S. (1972). Sex Education Symposium. *J Special Education* 5, 4, 351–81.

Gordon, S. (1973). *On being the Parent of a Handicapped Youth*. New York Association for Brain Injured Children and its Associations for Children with Learning Disabilities, 95 Madison Avenue, New York, NY 10016.

Gordon, S. (1975). Workshop. Sex Education for the Handicapped. In Bass, M.S. and Gelof, M. (eds), *Sexual Rights and Responsibilities of the Mentally Retarded.* Proceedings of the Conference of American Association on Mental Deficiency, Region IX, 1972. (Revised edition.)

Gostin, L. (1980). Sterilization and the Law. *Parents Voice 30,* 4, 16–17.

Greengross, W. (1976). *Entitled to Love.* London: Mallaby Press.

Grunewald, K. (1979). Sex Liberation and Parenthood for the Mentally Retarded in Sweden. Paper published by Socialstyrelsen, the National Board of Health and Welfare, 106 30 Stockholm, Sweden, July 1979.

Grunewald, K. and Linner, B. (1979). Mentally Retarded: Sexuality and Normalization. *Current Sweden* No 237, Dec. 1979.

Hall, J.E. (1974). Sexual Behavior. In: Wortis, J. (ed) *Mental Retardation (and Developmental Disabilities): An Annual Review.* Vol VI. New York: Brunner/Mazel.

Hall, J.E. (1975). Sexuality and the Mentally Retarded. In: Green, R. (ed) *Human Sexuality: A Health Practitioner's Text.* Baltimore: Williams and Wilkins.

Hall, J.E. (1978). Acceptance of Sexual Expression in the Mentally Retarded. *Sexuality and Disability 1,* 1, 44-51.

Hall, J.E. and Morris, H.L. (1976). Sexual Knowledge and Attitudes of Institutionalized and non-Institutionalized Adolescents. *Am.J.Ment.Defic.* 80,4, 382-7.

Hall, J.E., Morris, H.L. and Barker, H.R. (1973). Sexual Knowledge and Attitudes in Mentally Retarded Adolescents. *Am.J.Ment.Defic. 77,* 706-9.

Hall, J.E. and Sawyer, H.W. (1978). Sexual Policies for the Mentally Retarded. *Sexuality and Disability 1,* 1, 34-43.

Hammar, S.L., Wright, L.S. and Jensen, D.L. (1967). Sex Education for the Retarded Adolescent: A Survey of Parental Attitudes and Methods of Management in 50 Retarded Adolescents. *Clin. Pediatrics 6,* 621-7.

Hamre-Nietupski, S. and Ford, A. (1981). Sex Education and Related Skills: A Series of Programs Implemented with Severely Handicapped Students. *Sexuality and Disability 4,* 3, 179–93.

Hamre-Nietupski, S. and Williams, W. (1977) Implementation of Selected Sex Education and Social Skills to Severely Handicapped Students. *Education and Training of the Mentally Retarded 12,* 364-72.

Harris, A. (1974). What Does "Sex Education" Mean? In: Rogers, R. (ed) *Sex Education: Rationale and Reaction.* Cambridge: Cambridge University Press.

Hartman, S.S. and Hynes, J. (1975). Marriage Education for Mentally Retarded Adults. *Social Casework,* May, 280-4.

Hastings Center Report (1978). Sterilization of the Retarded: In Whose Interest? *8,* 3, 28-41.

Isaev, D.N. (1979). Learning About Sex. *World Health,* October, 20-3.

Johnson, W.R. (1973). Sex Education of the Mentally Retarded. In: de la Cruz,

F.F. and LaVeck, G.D. (eds) *Human Sexuality and the Mentally Retarded.* London: Butterworth.

Kempton, W. (1972). *Guidelines for Planning a Training Course on Human Sexuality and the Retarded.* Philadelphia: Planned Parenthood Association of South Eastern Pennsylvania.

Kempton, W. (1975). *A Teacher's Guide to Sex Education for Persons with Learning Disabilities.* North Scituate, Mass: Duxbury Press.

Kempton, W. (1976). Sexual Rights and Responsibilities of the Retarded Person. Official Proceedings of the 103rd Annual Social Welfare Forum. National Conference on Social Welfare, Washington, D.C., June 13-17, 1976. New York: Columbia University Press.

Kempton, W. (1977a). The Mentally Retarded Person. In: Gochros, H. and Gochros, J. (eds) *The Sexually Oppressed.* New York: Association Press.

Kempton, W. (1977b). The Sexual Adolescent who is Retarded. *J. Pediatric Psychology 2,* 3, 104–7.

Kempton W. (1978). Sex Education for the Mentally Handicapped. *Sexuality and Disability 1,* 2, 137–46.

Kempton, W. (1979). A Review of Intrauterine Devices. *Brit.J.Sexual Medicine 6,* 51, 16–17.

Kempton, W., Bass, M. and Gordon, S. (1972). *Love, Sex and Birth Control for the Mentally Retarded: A Guide for Parents.* Philadelphia: Planned Parenthood Association of South Eastern Pennsylvania.

Kempton, W. and Forman, R. (1976). *Guidelines for Training in Sexuality and the Mentally Handicapped.* Philadelphia: Planned Parenthood Association of South Eastern Pennsylvania.

Lee, G. (1976). *Sex Education and the Mentally Retarded.* London: National Society for Mentally Handicapped Children.

Lee, G. and Katz, G. (1974). *Sexual Rights of the Retarded.* London: National Society for Mentally Handicapped Children.

Livock, R. (1979). Developing a Sexual Policy. *Community Care,* 7 June, 22–3.

MacEachron, A.E. (1979). Mentally Retarded Offenders: Prevalence and Characteristics. *Am.J.Ment.Defic. 84,* 2, 165–76.

MacKenzie, N. and MacKenzie, J. (1977). *The First Fabians.* London: Weidenfeld and Nicolson.

MacLean, R. (1979). Sexual Problems and Family Planning Needs of the Mentally Handicapped in Residential Care. *Brit.J.Family Planning, 4,* 4, 13–15.

Mattinson, J. (1975). *Marriage and Mental Handicap.* 2nd editn. London: Institute of Marital Studies, The Tavistock Institute of Human Relations.

May, D.C. (1980). Survey of Sex Education Coursework in Special Education Programs. *J.Special Education 14,* 1, 107–12.

Meyen, E.L. (1970). Sex Education for the Mentally Retarded. Implications for programming and teacher training. *Focus on Exceptional Children 1,* 8, 1–5.

Meyen, E.L. and Retish, P.M. (1971). Sex Education for the Mentally Retarded: Influencing Teachers' Attitudes. *Ment.Retardation 9,* 46–9.

Meyerowitz, J.H. (1971). Sex and the Mentally Retarded. *Med.AspectsHum.Sexual 5,* 11, 94–118.

Mitchell, L.K., Doctor, R.M. and Butler, D.C. (undated). *A Manual for Behavioral Intervention on the Sexual Problems of Retarded Individuals in Residential or Home Settings.* Available from Dr L. Mitchell, Department of Counselor Education, California State University, Los Angeles, CA 90032, USA.

Mitchell, L.K., Doctor, R.M. and Butler, D.C. (1978). Attitudes of Caretakers towards the Sexual Behavior of Mentally Retarded Persons. *Am.J.Ment.Defic. 83,* 3, 289–96.

35

Mittler, P. (1979). Educating Mentally Handicapped Children. In: Craft, M. (ed) *Tredgold's Mental Retardation*, 12th editn. London: Balliere Tindall.

Mosier, H.D., Grossman, H.J. and Dingman, H.F. (1962). Secondary Sex Development in Mentally Deficient Individuals. *Child Development 33*, 273–86.

Mulhern, T.J. (1975). Survey of Reported Sexual Behavior and Policies Characterising Residential Facilities for Retarded Citizens. *Am.J.Ment.Defi. 79*, 6, 670–3.

National Development Group for the Mentally Handicapped (1980). *Improving the Quality of Services for Mentally Handicapped People: a Check List of Standards*. London: DHSS.

Parker, E. (1974). *Survey of Incapacity Associated with Mental Handicap at Rampton and Moss Side Special Hospitals*. Special Hospitals Research Report No. 11. Special Hospitals Research Unit.

Perske, R. (1972). The Dignity of Risk and the Mentally Retarded. *Ment.Retardation 10*, 1, 25–7.

Polvinale, R.A. and Lutzker, J.R. (1980). Elimination of Asaultative and Inappropriate Sexual Behavior by Reinforcement and Social Restitution. *Ment.Retardation 18*, 1, 27–30.

Reed, S.C. and Anderson, V.E. (1973). Effects of changing sexuality on the gene pool. In: de la Cruz, F.F. and LaVeck, G.D. (eds) *Human and Sexuality and the Mentally Retarded*. London: Butterworth.

Reed, E.W. and Reed, S.C. (1965). *Mental Retardation: A Family Study*. Philadelphia: Saunders.

Reich, M. and Harshman, H. (1971). Sex Education for Handicapped Youngsters, Reality or Repression? *J.Special Education 5*, 373–77.

Rosen, M. (1970). Conditioning Appropriate Heterosexual Behavior in Mentally and Socially Handicapped Populations. *Training School Bulletin 66*, 172–7.

Rosen, M. (1975). Psychosexual Adjustment of the Mentally Handicapped. In: Bass, M.S. and Gelof, M. (eds) *Sexual Rights and Responsibilities of the Mentally Retarded*. Proceedings of the Conference of American Association on Mental Deficiency, Region IX, 1972. (Revised editn.)

Salerno, L.J., Park, J.K. and Giannini, M.J. (1975). Reproductive Capacity of the Mentally Retarded. *J. Reproductive Medicine 14*, 3, 123–9.

Sandtner, E.S. (1972). Sexual Expectations of the Mentally Retarded. *Ment.Retardation 10*, 27–9.

Saunders, E.J. (1979). Staff Members' Attitudes towards the Sexual Behavior of Mentally Retarded Residents. *Am.J.Ment.Defic. 84*, 2, 206–8.

Scally, B.G. (1973). Marriage and Mental Retardation: some observations in Northern Ireland. In: de la Cruz, F.F. and LaVeck, G.D. (eds) (1973) *Human Sexuality and the Mentally Retarded*. New York: Brunner/Mazel; London: Butterworths.

Schofield, M. (1968). *A Study of the Sexual Behaviour of Young People*. Harmondsworth: Pelican.

Shaw, C.H. and Wright, C.H. (1960). The Married Mental Defective: A Follow-up Study. *Lancet 1*, 273–4.

Shennan, V. (1976). *Help your Child to Understand Sex*. London: National Society for Mentally Handicapped Children.

Shindell, P.E. (1975). Sex Education Programs and the Mentally Retarded. *J.School Health XLV*, 2, 88–90.

Special Education Curriculum Development Center (1972). *Social and Sexual Development: A guide for teachers of the handicapped*. Revised edition. University of Iowa, Iowa City, Iowa 52242, USA.

Terman, L. (1916). *The Measurement of Intelligence*. Boston: Houghton Mifflin Co.

Tricomi, V., Valenti, C. and Hall, J.E. (1964). Ovulatory Pattern in Down's Syndrome. *Am.J.Obstet.Gynec. 89,* 651–6.

United Nations (1971). *Declaration of General and Special Rights of the Mentally Handicapped.* New York; UN Department of Social Affairs.

Walker, N. and McCabe, S. (1973). *Crime and Insanity in England.* Vol. 2. Edinburgh: University Press.

Watson, G. (1980). Sex Education Surveyed. *Special Education, Forward Trends 7,* 3, 11–14.

Watson, G. and Rogers, R.S. (1980). Sexual Instruction for the Mildly Retarded and Normal Adolescent: A comparison of educational approaches, parental expectations and pupil knowledge and attitude. *Health Education Journal 39,* 3, 88–95.

Whittemore, R.D. and Koegal, P. (1978). *Loving Alone is not Helpful: Sexuality and social context among the mildly retarded.* Working Paper 7, Socio-Behavioral Group, Mental Retardation Research Center, School of Medicine, University of California, Los Angeles, USA.

Wilson, R.R. and Baldwin, B.A. (1976). A Pilot Sexuality Training Workshop for Staff at an Institution for the Mentally Retarded. *Am.J.Public Health 66,* 77–78.

Wish, J.R., McCombs, K.F. and Edmonson B. (1980). *The Socio-Sexual Knowledge and Attitude Test.* Stoelting Company, 1350 S Kostner Ave., Chicago, Ill. 70623, USA.

Wolfensberger, W. (1972). *The Principle of Normalization in Human Services.* Toronto, Canada: National Institute on Mental Retardation.

Wright, S.W., Tarjan, G. and Eyer, L. (1959). Investigation of families with two or more mentally defective siblings. *Am.J.Dis.Child.* 97, 445–63.

CHAPTER 2

Sexual Behaviour and Sexual Difficulties

Michael Craft

Traditionally, sexual expression by mentally retarded members of Western society has been suspect—giving rise to anxiety for any one or combination of reasons (the list is by no means exhaustive):

(a) By virtue of the mental handicap *per se.*
(b) The possible unwanted consequences (pregnancy, bad reputation for the residential unit).
(c) The behaviour is illegal.
(d) The behaviour is seen as immoral.
(e) It is potentially dangerous (to the subject or partner).
(f) It is inappropriate (place, partner or frequency).

Parents and care-givers alike are often very unclear in their thinking about sexual expression, and therefore in their responses to it. Is a particular behaviour a stage of "normal" human development, or does it warrant "treatment"? Either way the behaviour is highly likely to be seen as a "problem" by those who have responsibility for the care of the retarded individual.

What is "Normal"?

Much of the confusion springs from the different meanings of the word *normal.* We use different models of normality in different contexts, and in doing so often confuse ourselves and everyone else. Johnson (1975) identifies five models of normality.

The *subjective* model is probably best summed up in the Quaker saying: "All the world's queer save thee and me, and even thee is a little queer". Kinsey *et al.* (1948) found that men generally considered their own frequency of masturbation to be normal, be it once a day or once a month, but thought that greater frequency had ill effects, and less frequency indicated a degree of sexual inadequacy.

The *moral* model. Within this model abnormality equates with sin. The traditional criteria of normal sexual relations in our society has been the man's penis fitting inside the woman's vagina, using the missionary position, ideally aimed at reproduction, all taking place in the context of marriage. By traditional standards of sexual morality many people are immoral, but the standard has to be taken seriously because the laws regarding sexual offence generally derive from it. While large segments of the population may view recreational sex in its various forms as entirely normal, the law does not tend to do so. Nor do most parents or most officials associated with the law, with education, with hospitals or institutions where traditional morality tends to dictate sexual normality. In America, the Institute for Sex Research recently conducted a national survey which found that the majority of adults are strongly opposed to homosexuality and adultery and do not accept premarital coitus even between adults (Gebhard 1980). The statistical model (below) reveals a different picture.

The *cultural* model. Anthropological studies have revealed an enormous range in what different societies call normal and abnormal sexual behaviour (Marshall and Suggs 1971). Many nineteenth century travellers and missionaries made very firm judgments about the immorality of other societies on the basis of their own cultural model. In ancient Greece it was said, "A boy for pleasure, a woman for business"; twentieth century Pathans from Afghanistan added to this, "A goat for preference".

Within the cultural model, there are of course variations for different racial and socio-economic groups. Arranged marriages, for instance, conflict with the western model of dating, courtship and personal choice, but they remain a feature of Indian and Pakistani immigrant communities in Britain. There is a strong case for postulating that mentally handicapped people in hospitals and colonies have evolved essentially adaptive sexual behaviours in response to their particular institutional subculture (Rosen 1975). We know that most behaviours are learned as a result of personal experience and environmental influences. We also know that institutions, whatever their formal aims, tend not to be settings which promote behaviour that would be considered normal in the community at large. Indeed, the reverse seem to happen (Bouliew 1971). Staff have often been conditioned to expect and excuse behaviour which would be seen as illegal, immoral, ludicrous or weird beyond the gates. The normality of certain behaviours within the institution, for example homosexual contacts, exposure of male genitalia, public stripping, groping and clinging, is in direct contradition to the wider cultural model of normality, and certainly to the moral model. As in many other areas of life, we operate on double or even treble standards.

The *statistical* model. Abnormality is here a deviation from the mean. This model is comparatively recent with regard to sexual behaviour. Kinsey and his colleagues (1948 and 1953) were among the first to compile statistics on sexual expression. It is important to remember that the Kinsey findings only held true for white middle-class Americans in the 1940s. The statistical model is often at variance with the other models, particularly the moral one. For example, Kinsey showed that a surprisingly large percentage, over one third, of the 4,000 American whites on his survey had had adult homosexual experience over the age of 16. Some ten per cent continued homosexual practice within and without marriage in their adult years. Kinsey *et al.* 1948 and 1953 further showed that masturbation is very common sexual behaviour. According to Gebbard (1980) its frequency over the past few decades has changed little. While there has always been an almost one hundred per cent incidence among males, there has been an increase in females to at least the two-thirds level. The statistical model helps to demonstrate trends and changes which are taking place in sexual behaviour. The Kinsey date revealed that eight per cent of females born before 1900 had had premarital coitus by age 20 (Kinsey *et al.* 1948, 1953), and this percentage gradually rose until among women born between 1910 and 1919 some 23 per cent had had premarital coitus by age 20. In 1967 a study by the American Institute for Sex Research showed that 33 per cent of the unmarried college females on their study were no longer virgins by age 20. Later studies show an increase in incidence of premarital sexual intercourse (Gebhard 1980). Adultery committed by men seems to have changed little in incidence from the 1940s to the present day, hovering between 40 and 50 per cent. However, adultery has increased among females. The Kinsey figure of 26 per cent has now risen to 36 per cent, according to Athanasiou *et al.* (1970).

The *clinical* model. This equates normality with health and health-promoting behaviour, so the unhappy, the unsatisfied, the anxious and those feeling themselves inadequate are abnormal.

Becoming normal may well clash with other models, so that the unmarried person pursuing a sex life contravenes the moral model.

Psychosexual Development

Psychosexual development starts before birth, for at conception both the sex chromosomes are established which visibly set the individual towards his or her sexual identity at birth. Thereafter, the normal baby achieves bonding with its mother, or mother substitute, learning the enjoyment of love, cuddling, fondling and bodily comfort. In addition, the normal baby is physically stimulated by the development of what Freud called the erogenous zones, firstly of mouth, then anus and finally of genitals. Quite young baby boys can respond with an erection to the stimulation of their own genitals, and some learn to do this themselves from the age of one with obvious relief when they complete what appears to be a climax. These twin developments are a feature of childhood, so that while growing the child continues to enjoy maternal and paternal love during the school years, he is also learning that there are degrees of loving, cuddling and bodily enjoyment appropriate to different types of human relationship. At school there is both the enjoyment of one's own bodily sensations as a result of physical activity and the physical contact with other humans. Each have different emotional impacts dependent on the excitation of the situations under which they are enjoyed. Both these sets of feelings are predominantly learned behavioural responses, so that the child whose natural mother hands it to a foster or adoptive mother may have an entirely satisfactory loving relationship with that substitute mother, learning to cuddle, to be comforted and to comfort, to tell her that he loves her, and to receive a great deal of loving enjoyment in return.

Having successfully learned both to receive and to give such love, the normally developing child will be able to transfer this learned experience to others, and develop satisfactory relationships with children and later adolescents in the course of his or her school career. The deprived child may not learn such love. Lacking tuition in love from a cold mother who has failed to bond to her child, or more commonly a foster or adoptive mother who fails to establish a true bond, this child may grow up egocentric, emotionally cold, or emotionally uncertain. The over-mothered child may develop an abnormal response. Here too the "smothered" child, perhaps the product of a single parent, or a mother herself emotionally deprived, may grow up expecting to be given all and to give nothing in return, a variation on the egocentric model noted above. This child may be called "emotionally immature" in the sense that the emotional relationship is all one way. Perhaps more common is the child with an emotionally unstable mother, who himself develops swings of emotional moods and of capacity to love.

In an imperfect world with so many imperfect parents, the wonder of it is to the psychiatric writer, that so many humans turn out to be remarkably loving, when their developmental patterns have been so abysmal. The odds are strongly in favour of the well-loved child developing into a loving adult, but the resilience of human nature is such that many unloved children still have considerable capacities for loving behaviour if environmental circumstances go in their favour at a later date.

So much for the development of loving ability. Physical stimulation to orgasm has a number of more mechanical features which allow a climax to be reached by a baby boy less than one year old. Because the erogenous genital zone of a female is better protected, baby girls generally do not learn the physical ability to masturbate to climax as early as boys, although there are well recorded instances of self-induced orgasm before schooling at five. Physical stimulation or orgasm as a learned experience obviously depends for its use and its frequency on competing occupations of infancy and childhood, so that the child busy with hands, toys or other interests is least likely to become centred on stimulation of its own private parts. There is one other highly important feature in this area to which attention must be drawn. Probably as a result of evolutionary pressures, humans, like other animals, have developed enhanced abilities to respond to extreme emotions. The secretion of internal hormones, such as adrenalin, at times of fright or flight heightens the swiftness of response of the alerted animal, and also activates an enhancement of memory recall for the situation involved. This enhancement of memory is due to a second biochemical feature in animals, a neurotransmitter mechanism within the brain which increases the depth of memory of strongly emotional responses, and increases the speed of recall. Thus a severe fright greatly sensitizes the human response to other frights of similar character, even to the stage where an over-reaction—a

42

panic state—ensues. While self physical stimulation by masturbation is not likely to lead to any strong emotional response, a seduction or rape is most likely to do so, although not the seduction of a child by another child of similar age. It is a frightening seduction by an older person, or the fear of a recurrence of an actual childhood rape which produces a strong emotional response. Childhood sexual experiences are not that uncommon, adolescent boys are very likely to sexually experiment with their own sex at puberty, and some enjoy such an emotional heightening of their first climaxes that they never wish to experiment in any other way, conditioning themselves to respond preferentially in this way for the rest of their lives. This may be one explanation for the fact that some adult males persist in their attempts to gain sexual climax with small boys, pubescent boys or adolescent boys; but it cannot be the only reason, for most adolescent boys experiment in this way, and only a small minority persist. Far fewer adolescent girls complete their first climaxes with each other, but as with boys, the first sexual experience of a woman is usually highly important for her.

The father, as well as the mother, has an important part to play in the normal psychosexual development of the child. The main role of the father is in teaching the developing child love by example. By his shown love to mother, by his care of both, he teaches the developing child a pattern of the loving relationship between an adult man and women by acting as a model in this respect as in others. During childhood he has a principal part to place in the setting of bounds, those limits of behaviour beyond which the child is conditioned not to go. Each culture has its different values and bounds to be set, with regard to sexual behaviour. Western culture disapproves of children exposing their genitals, engaging in excessive open sexual violence and using verbal sexual obscenities. During adolescence the ideal father teaches his son factual knowledge concerning sexual conduct and norms of courtship, and may still set bounds by conditioning and using disciplinary procedures and penalties (adolescent girls ideally learn from their mothers).

There are also a wide variety of mislearning situations that fathers can inculcate. From Henry Williamson's *Donkey Boy* comes the painful lesson from father that sex is something "dirty" or "not nice":

Letting himself into the house with his latchkey, quietly [Phillip's father] had heard the children playing in the front room; and looking round the half-open door, to give them a surprise, he had been shocked by what he had seen. There was Phillip under the table, struggling with Mavis and interfering with her clothes. Dickie heard Phillip saying, "Come on, be fair, I have shown you mine, now you must show me yours!" Hauling him in a rage from under the table by a leg, Richard had set the boy on his feet, and demanded to know what he meant by it.

"Nothing, Father."

"I'll teach you to behave like that, you disgusting little beast! How dare you?"

He had shaken Phillip, hit him with his flat hand on the side of the head, then put him across his knee, and holding him with one hand by the neck, beaten him as hard as he could with his other hand. Afterwards, Phillip had been sent upstairs to bed.

Other mislearning experiences may become the financial reward of prostitutes and the despair of wives. Whips, scourges, chains, ropes and other materials bear testimony to the exquisite emotional memories of earlier sexual experiences in aiding many remarkably well educated men to achieve their climax. The repeated newspaper reports of judges, peers of the realm and other talented people who need to pay for their sexual climaxes in this way, make it quite clear that with some, early learned experiences can condition them for life. Other conditioning experiences lie behind varietes of fetishism or pedophilia.

The discussion above has been mainly in terms of the development of normal members of society. The mentally handicapped are much more likely to have a less normal type of upbringing. Down's syndrome people who comprise one third of the severely handicapped are commonly born to elderly parents at the end of both their reproductive and working careers. They are far more likely to have the undivided attention of mother to protect, and father to safeguard them from peril, than older siblings, who therefore have both more time and opportunity to learn about the risks of life in sexual as in other spheres. Although the mentally handicapped have an age of menarche and puberty not too dissimilar to the norm, they are much more likely to be smothered by care and to have fewer opportunities than normal siblings, either of developing an adult relationship with their peer group, or for that matter of being able to settle down in a constructive partnership. Thus the stresses and strains of learned experiences in the sexual field are different for the mentally handicapped, and to analyse these the professional needs knowledge of normal development against which to evaluate the problem of the handicapped, and a framework of reference so that he knows where to start to analyse what might have gone wrong.

Sexual Dysfunction and Sexual Deviation

Over the last twenty years the studies of Kinsey and his colleagues (1948 and 1953), and Masters and Johnson (1966, 1970 and 1979) have advanced our understanding of the complexity of "normal" sexuality among normal people, also our understanding of what can go wrong with sexual function. But all treatment costs money and resources, and is expanded to suit the demands of the population at risk. Until quite recently the normal population, although articulate, educated and monied when compared with their grandparents, did not demand help for sexual problems, although such problems presumably have been manifest in each generation. One only has to contrast the articles appearing in the women's magazines of today with those of twenty years ago to appreciate that there has been a shift in sexual expectations. We are still only slowly coming to terms with that shift, and seeing and responding to sexual dysfunction in the same way as any other disorder of the human condition.

In analyses of normal populations, sexual difficulties are usually divided into sexual dysfunction and sexual deviation. Dysfunction describes the situation where the male or female experiences an absolute or relative deficit in sexual performance. These deficits may spring from a variety of causes, both organic and psychiatric. Sexual deviation is at once simple, yet hard to define, for it is merely a list of sexual behaviours which are unacceptable to a given culture. Yet acceptable sexual practices may contain elements which if extreme would be classed as deviant—mildly sadistic behaviour is not uncommon, although infliction of humiliation and much physical pain on a sexual partner is considered abnormal in western society (Bebbington 1979). Disorders of sexual orientation in this culture would include homosexuality, pedophilia, exhibitionism, voyerism, sadomasochism, frotteurism, fetishism and others such as bestiality and necrophilia. Gender role abnormalities, such as transvestism or transexualism are often classed as sexual deviations.

Dysfunction and Deviation in the Retarded Person

Not surprisingly, as the weight of opinion has traditionally been against *any* sexual function by those labelled mentally handicapped, literature on their sexual dysfunction is practically non-existent. It has not yet attracted research, and it is not a condition about which many of the handicapped themselves complain.*

That is not to say that retarded persons do not experience the same kinds of sexual dysfunction as the normal population (Chapter 12 clearly indicates that they do). It is just that in general we are not so good at identifying or treating them. One dysfunction which is receiving attention is the failure to masturbate to orgasm, usually found in severely mentally handicapped individuals, although Rosen (1970) mentions this in connection with some mildly retarded sex offenders.

The distinction between sexual dysfunction and sexual deviation cannot be so firmly drawn when the population at issue is retarded, because of the develomental delays. A normal toddler has learned how comforting can be his mother's lap and human touch and caress. What of the physically large 16 year old autistic boy slowly discovering the warmth and good feeling involved in touch, who clings to care staff? His normal peers have probably moved through a homosexual phase, and are busily experimenting with heterosexual contact, so our autistic boy may be said to have a deficit in sexual performance—dysfunction. If the staff he clings to happen to be male, someone is bound to talk in terms of homosexual behaviour—sexual deviation. Neither is really appropriate to describe what is going on.

But what is it that is going on? A normal, but delayed psychosexual developmental phase or a learned and purposive behaviour which is usually successful at gaining the now desired goal of attention? Probably a combination of both. While we recognise the normality of the phase, we need to channel behaviour along more appropriate lines. It is common for normal humans at various stages in their lives to enjoy nakedness, to get pleasure out of touching their genitalia, to be proud of an exposed and erect penis,

* Personal experience indicates that where retarded married couples experience what *objectively* might be classed as sexual dysfunction, it may not *subjectively* be counted as such, perhaps because expectations are low. There are, of course, many marriages between normal people for which this is also true.

46

and to receive a degree of sexual stimulation, either from tickling others or being tickled, together with energetic physical play and body contact. Homosexual play seems far more common among pubescent males than among pubescent females, although after puberty the sexes normally get a great deal of pleasure from each other and pairing (usually of a temporary nature) becomes a feature of adolescent human activity.

Thus by two or three of the models of normality the enjoyment of exhibitionism, voyeurism, homosexuality and heterosexual crushes are by no means abnormal, although they may contravene the cultural and moral models. Difficulties may arise for mentally handicapped people because they fail to grasp that the "normal" adults around them use the variety of "double talk" in the field of sexual behaviour. The subtleties involved in "do as I say, not do as I do" often pass the mentally handicapped person by, with the result that they overstep boundaries of behaviour.

We have seen how hard normality is to define and we are a long way from possessing adequate knowledge about the psychosexual development patterns of retarded persons (Chapter 10 examines many of the complexities involved). We know from Kinsey's work that about four per cent of male subjects were exclusively homosexual, ten per cent in all were more or less exclusively homosexual (1948). Of the female subjects surveyed, four per cent were exclusively lesbian between the ages of 20 to 55 (1955). Sexual deviations, however, represent only a fraction of the total population, and this is probably true also of the retarded as well as the normal. According to Gebhard (1980), speaking of the American scene, homosexual activity and deviations such as fetishism and sadomasochism seem largely independent of social change. That is to say they have not increased in recent decades. This would seem to indicate a more or less constant proportion of such men and women, stable over time. It is harder to quantify for those we label "mentally handicapped" because of their segregated living circumstances, and lack of opportunities for normal learning experiences. There is certainly a small proportion of men who show a persisting and unswerving interest in only members of their own sex, paying no attention to females either during puberty or adulthood.

Many more are situationally homosexual, but this may only be discovered by chance. When men from a monosexual unit in Wales were moved to a new hospital opening for both sexes, many thought to be confirmed homosexuals over many years confounded staff by switching their attention to the lady residents, often displaying much charm and no little social skill. The "problems" they then presented were of a different order!

Analysing the Sexual Difficulties of the Mentally Handicapped Individual

Clearly, the professional faced with the request to examine a mental retarded person ostensibly having sexual difficulties needs a frame of reference within which to work. The previous part of this chapter has afforded a background of what to expect with normal humans, together with the special modifications needed to this framework to allow for the retardate's slow mental development but almost normal physical development. The model of analysis now to be presented can be used by any professional with time and sympathy to spare, but it is worthwhile noting that a doctor could bring three elements to bear on the situation over and above other professionals. Firstly, from a physical examination he might detect abnormalities such as a tight prepuce, vaginal inflamation, or urinary irritation due to undiagnosed diabetes; secondly, on mental examination he could diagnose a superimposed mental illness such as schizophrenia; and thirdly, he can prescribe drugs for any of the above should these be necessary. Despite this, the vast majority of sexual difficulties are within the compass of the non-medical professional to investigate and help.

Primary sexual difficulties are rarely complained about by the retarded person. The difficulties in obtaining an erection at the proper time, holding it, or effecting ejaculation which so beset modern man, are less likely to be a worry to the retardate, because he does not have access to the literature and media presentation to the same extent as the ordinary adult male. The misdirection of sexual desire, such as homosexuality or bestialism is likely to be complained about by the mentally handicapped individual only when he has been caught out and punished for it. It is important to obtain the retarded person's view on the subject about which there is complaint, because his version may provide the diagnostic clue. Tight pants or irritation or provocation by a third party, may not have been revealed to an aggrieved teacher seen predominantly in a

48

disciplinary capacity. Discussion with the individual on his own in his bedroom, where he feels most at ease, may also allow him to explain what he wants out of the sexual situation. The shy mentally handicapped person often has difficulty in expressing his feelings towards a third party, male or female, or the provocation which may have ensued as a result of chance features. From such an interview, the writer discovered that a 20 year old Down's syndrome man was being rewarded by cigarettes and sweets for his excessive masturbation by an older fellow resident sleeping in the same bedroom in the hostel. In the under-staffed hostel, the warden had early taken a disciplinary stance and had never elicited the true facts of the situation before calling for supressant drugs and removal of the offender.

By *secondary sexual difficulties* is meant the agitation, distress and secondary mental disturbance that are evinced by the individual in difficulty. Particularly with the retarded, these may be the main feature of the situation, with aggression, verbal abuse, sleeplessness or staff-mauling being the main features behind the complaint. That unrelieved sexual tension causes difficulties to normal people in our society is now well recognized, but it is less well recognized that the same features may affect the mentally handicapped as well, particularly in late teens at the height of their particular sexual drive. Behind this tension may also be the drive towards the retarded person's concept of "normality", and in this he is as open to stimulation by television and advertisements as anybody else. Retarded people are as capable of "bonding" as other members of society, so that in the common situation where a delinquent mildly mentally handicapped boy is admitted to a hostel because of his offences, the collusion of his family, and general mayhem in his home area; his seduction of a severely handicapped girl more normally brought up may be as much a tragedy for her as for other members of society deprived of someone they love. Thus weeping, sleeplessness, attacks on staff, smashing and general destruction after being jilted, may be explainable as a positive feature of her ability to 'bond' even if it was initially to the wrong boy at the wrong time, who has now departed. Once explained in this way to harrassed staff, they may be considerably more sympathetic, especially as the experience would be common to them as well. With the retarded girl, just as with others, such an experience may be suppressed for some months before coming into the open. For fear

49

of parental disapproval or staff disciplinary action, she may have hidden her true feelings for as long as she was able to, thus mystifying staff and causing a misunderstanding when she finally 'breaks down'. It is a truism to say that the more normally the mentally handicapped person has been brought up, the more he or she is capable of this type of tension display, for a child who has not been taught to love is less likely to bond, and less likely to be affected by the departure of staff or resident to whom he or she had taken a fancy. The much-moved adolescent passed on from home to home has a far more callous view of things and his sexual tension is much more likely to be displayed in a calculated outburst and display of rage or aggression to get at the things he needs right then to secure his goal.

The tertiary level of sexual dysfunction is that which causes its main effect on third parties who themselves bring the complaint. For example, a homosexual retarded male may be content with his own direction of sex drive, and thoroughly enjoying the results, but give cause for complaint by the young boys whom he takes, or the staff who have to bear the responsibility. In such a situation, it is sometimes possible for staff members to counsel the man and aid him to follow the direction of his sexual desire with a suitable adult partner who can legally give valid consent. A case conference of staff may be necessary, to allow dissenting staff members to air their views, and formulate a concerted policy on the subject, but if the examining professional persuades them that this kind of pairing can have a constructive value, in the sense of relief of tension, enjoyment of company and humane behaviour, the conference may have achieved its object.

At other times it may be the staff themselves who are over zealous. One hostel called the writer to suppress 'grossly abnormal behaviour patterns' with a 44 year old mildly retarded man who was busily seducing a 24 year old mildly retarded female morning, noon and night. They had been banished to different parts of the same hostel but still found opportunity to hold hands beneath the dining room table, to disappear into the bushes at the back of the hostel at washing up time, or to indulge in unseemly behaviour in the darkened television room. During the complete history-taking, it was established that the couple themselves were very happy, although indeed their 'grossly abnormal behaviour patterns' were abnormal so far as the rules of the hostel were concerned. More

50

relevant was the fury of the hostel warden, herself going through a divorce because her husband had seduced a younger woman and was busily consorting with her morning, noon and night. The rules of the Social Service Department do not allow intercourse in hostels, nor would they allow the suggested solution: marriage and married quarters. It was not possible to transfer the couple to another unit because of the disapproval of the Director of Social Services to this 'grossly abnormal behaviour'. They were finally admitted to hospital, not because they needed treatment, but because it was the only place willing to supply both the married accommodation and the level of daily support the couple needed. Following counselling they married, and settled down together. The couple were eventually placed out in a bed sitting room on a country estate, working as subsidised domestic worker and gardener and remain happy and content.

The *staff case conference* can be a very constructive way of approaching some of the difficulties described above. Apart from gaining more than one account of the situation complained about, interaction among staff members allows the examining professional to make a better evaluation of the developing situation and ways forward. Sympathetic staff can be supported and encouraged, the legal position clarified and a consensus will often emerge. The full staff conference may also allow other methods to succeed. A typewritten report of a conference, with copies to those concerned, is an effective way of publicizing united viewpoints, and bringing pressure to bear upon administrators and managers. The risks of sexual activity often provoke considerable emotional feeling among those peripherally involved, and particularly where knowledge is scanty and one or two stages removed from the situation, directives from above may be laid down which have little regard for individual feelings. For the unhappy residential care worker who knows that what he is commanded to do is wrong in theory as well as in practice, it may be of little help to advise education at all levels. Other chapters in this book examine the risks involved in sexual activity, and the contentious issues of birth control, sterilization and marriage, for after all it was the need for education and evaluation which prompted this book being written in the first place. Where education is insufficient, publication in local or professional journal, pressure groups inside and outside the orgnization may help, even the co-operative reporter of the local newspaper may be needed.

Conclusion

Sexual difficulties in the retarded are likely to be as common as in the normal person, although there has been little research in this area. This chapter has explored the pattern of growth of love and sexual ability in the normal person in order to provide background to the elucidation of difficulties in the retarded. In the last resort, simple explanations, education at a level which mentally handicapped people can understand, and the demonstration that loving can benefit all will do much to settle them and alleviate the worries of those who care for them.

REFERENCES

Athanasiou, R., Shaver, P. and Tavris, C. (1970). Sex. *Psychology Today 4*, 39–52.

Bebbington, P. (1979). Sexual Disorders. In: Hill, P., Murray, R. and Thorley, A. (eds). *Essentials of Postgraduate Psychiatry*. London: Academic Press.

Bouliew, D. (1971). Do Institutions Maintain Retarded Behavior? *Ment. Retardation 9*, 36–8.

Gebhard, P.H. (1980). Sexuality in the Post-Kinsey Era. In: Armytage, H.G., Chester, R. and Peel, J. (eds). *Changing Patterns of Sexual Behaviour*. London: Academic Press.

Johnson, W.R. (1975). *Sex Education and Counseling of Special Groups*. Springfield, Ill. : Charles C. Thomas.

Kinsey, A.C., Pomeroy, W.B. and Martin, C.E. (1948). *Sexual Behavior in the Human Male*. Philadelphia: Saunders.

Kinsey, A.C., Pomeroy, W.B., Martin, C.E. and Gebhard, P.H. (1953). *Sexual Behavior in the Human Female*. Philadelphia: Saunders.

Marshall, D.S. and Suggs, R.C. (1971). *Human Sexual Behavior*. New York: Basic Books.

Masters, W.H. and Johnson, V.E. (1966). *Human Sexual Response*. Boston: Little, Brown and Co.

Masters, W.H. and Johnson, V.E. (1970). *Human Sexual Inadequacy*. Boston: Little, Brown and Co.

Masters, W.H. and Johnson, V.E. (1979). *Homosexuality in perspective*. Boston: Little, Brown and Co.

Rosen, M. (1970). Conditioning Appropriate Heterosexual Behavior in Mentally and Socially Handicapped Populations. *Training School Bulletin 66*, 172–7.

Rosen, M. (1975). Psychosexual Adjustment of the Mentally Handicapped. In : Bass, M.S. and Gelof, M. (eds). *Sexual Rights and Responsibilities of the Mentally Retarded*. Proceedings of the Conference of American Association on Mental Deficiency, Region IX, 1972 (revised editition).

Williamson, H. (1962). *Donkey Boy*. St Albans: Panther Books.

CHAPTER 3

Sexuality Training for Professionals who Work with Mentally Handicapped Persons

Winifred Kempton

A programme for professionals to be trained to deal effectively with the sexuality of mentally handicapped persons is different from any other training; it is greatly challenging because it combines two of the most emotional aspects of living, sex and mental handicap. The three components of the training are: the subject matter, the mentally handicapped, and the trainees; all need special handling. First, the subject matter of sex is more emotion-packed then any other topic. Second, society has traditionally attempted to deny and repress the sexuality of mentally handicapped people, consequently, concepts on dealing with the reality of their sexual needs are vague and controversial. Third, the trainees, like *all* people have varying degrees of retardation when it comes to sexuality, and almost everyone has been sexually traumatized in one way or another. Thus, training is especially complicated and needs special procedures.

Training for work in most other fields usually involves presenting factual information, suggesting resources, teaching techniques, and polishing the skills of the trainees. These procedures are also important in sexuality training. However, not much can be accomplished unless the participants experience some of the special aspects of sexuality training such as: dispelling myths and misconceptions about sexuality often harboured from early childhood; relieving deep seated guilt feelings about being sexual; examining attitudes concerning controversial issues involving sexuality (especially concerning the mentally handicapped); developing comfort and confidence to enable them to discuss sexual topics for effective work in the trainees' own settings.

Training in sexuality and mental handicap is additionally complicated because it must deal with a wide span of attitudes and knowledge among the participants, and then must meet individual

53

needs. Additionally, the mentally handicapped to whom the training is addressed have widely differing abilities, ranging from those who can only learn the fundamentals of self-care and communication to those whose handicaps are so mild they cannot easily be discerned. These wide variations must be considered and matched with the needs of the trainees accordingly. Another special characteristic of sexuality training is that it must take into consideration the sexual politics existing in the trainees' work sites and their respective communities, where attitudes towards sexuality are often negative and/or highly controversial. The trainees need preparation for overcoming these barriers so they will be able to apply what they have learned after completing the course.

Considering all these complications it would seem that planning a training programme for professionals to deal with the sexuality of the mentally handicapped population is a mammoth task. However, in some parts of the world this training is being conducted, with exciting results. Although there is little research of the results of training programmes, first hand accounts of how training has been successfully used by graduates has given us enough confidence to present general guidelines that trainers can use in most settings where mentally handicapped persons are being taught, trained, or counselled. A brief description of these guidelines follows. It is recommended, however, that this information be supplemented by the book, *Guidelines For Training in Sexuality and the Mentally Handicapped* (Kempton and Forman, 1980) by the author of this chapter, based on her personal experiences while conducting dozens of training courses in most parts of the United States. The book contains a detailed description of topics that should be introduced in training, tests, resources available, and practical exercises that can be used for developing the skills of course participants.

Who Shall Be Trained?

Another way that training in sexuality and mental handicap differs from other training is that, when an agency or institution launches a sexuality programme controversy often arises as to whom shall be trained. Because the topic of sexuality threatens so many people, the idea of training can result in an anxious staff, divided in their opinions and feelings. Some are eager but frustrated because of

54

their lack of training; some will insist training is not needed and will be disinterested or resistant. Actually, everyone, without exception, needs some education, training, or guidance in dealing with the sexual behaviour of their mentally handicapped clients. This includes members of the administrative as well as the professional and supportive staffs. The educational needs of the staff may vary according to their duties and previous training; however, it is predictable that few staff members at any level of learning have received adequate training in the area of sexuality and that their attitudes will vary as much as their educational gaps. The goals of training an entire staff can be catergorized as follows:

Administrators need some exposure to sexuality education and training so that they will understand what is involved and the importance of including it in their overall programme. Since they are ultimately responsible they should be prepared to give their staff encouragement, support, and some guidance.

Professional Staff—Physicians, nurses, teachers, social workers, psychologists, psychiatrists, and counsellors need training because they may be mainly responsible for implementing education or sexuality counselling programmes. At the least, they should be prepared to deal with the problems that may arise from the sexual behaviour of the residents. They should supervise the direct care staff.

Attendant or Care Staff—The aides who have daily contact with mentally handicapped persons and who are responsible for the practical aspects of their care need to be prepared to deal with sexual behaviour as easily as with other behaviour, and especially to be mutually consistent in their attitudes and actions.

Supportive Staff—Office workers, maintenance and security staff, kitchen personnel, and volunteers, should be acquainted with their agencies' policies and be given enough orientation so that they will know what is expected of them. Otherwise, they may cause problems by well-meaning, but misdirected efforts to control (or encourage) inappropriate behaviour in the residents.

Although all staff members should be oriented to agency or institutional policies dealing with sexuality and have some understanding of resolving simple problems of sexuality, there should be a selected few persons designated to assume primary responsibility for counselling and teaching clients. Training for these professionals should be intensive and thorough either by their attendance at special workshops or university courses in sexuality, or both. These designated professionals should be interested in the subject of sexuality, and well motivated to assume the role of sex educators or counsellors. Randomly appointing staff members for these roles is not recommended; there are enough barriers to overcome during the training without having to deal with apathy or resistance from the trainees (during a training course it takes only a short time for the trainer to separate the participants who were *told* to attend from those who *asked* to take the course).

Obviously it would not be possible to offer this intensive training to an entire staff. However, planning an orientation programme or short-term training should include as many of the same components as intensive courses. Therefore, regardless of the time allowed for the training, whether three hours or three months, training in sexuality should include:

(1) presenting some factual information (especially to correct misinformation)
(2) exploring attitudes and attempting to improve the participant's comfort level in discussing the subject matter
(3) introducing the available techniques and resources
(4) pointing out the special needs and characeristics of mentally handicapped persons
(5) suggesting practical application of all of these

Testing and evaluation should be included in the training process. Tests help both trainer and participants to determine what knowledge and attitudes the group already possess and what needs are still to be met. Tests are available on attitudes towards sexuality in general and toward that of the mentally handicapped; on the factual apects of sexuality and reproduction; on the sexuality of the mentally handicapped; on venereal disease; on birth control. There are also tests to be given to the mentally handicapped themselves. Samples of these tests are contained in Kempton and Forman's Guide (1980), but others could be developed. *Evaluation questionnaires* for the trainees to answer at the end of their training have double values:

(1) their answers can be a valuable aid to the trainers in planning future courses, and

(2) participants can see what they have accomplished by the end of their training experience

Course Content

There are topics of almost universal interest and value for intensive training courses. Some topics can be introduced in separate sessions that stand on their own; however, some of the desired ultimate goals of developing personal comfort and sensitivity may be missed if the material is presented as separate entities. If a shorter course is all that is possible, a trainer will have to decide whether it is better to cover most of the topics briefly or to eliminate entirely those of lesser importance to the participants.

The remainder of this chapter will consist of brief descriptions of some important aspects of training, allowing much room for the creative ideas of the trainer. For clarity the topics will be described in the context of sessions.

Session I   Introducing the Participants to the Training Course

An important task in any programme involving sexuality is to establish a comfortable feeling among the participants; the trainer should try to do so as soon as possible. There are many methods to accomplish congeniality; entire books on "how to" exist. The method used depends on the trainer's preference, time allowed, size of the group, and the physical arrangements of the room. A place where chairs can be easily arranged, a rug and pillows (allowing the participants the choice of sitting on the floor) and enough space for mingling is highly preferable to a small, formal, lecture room.

Goals for this introductory part of the training are to help each participant to:
(1) feel comfortable as a member of the group
(2) have an understanding of why he or she is there, what to expect, and what the course will pursue
(3) develop a conviction of the need for sex education and counselling for the mentally handicapped, and
(4) alleviate doubts and anxieties about the results of such programmes

Training can proceed much more smoothly after these four goals are achieved. It is wise to dispel myths about sex education by holding a frank discussion on participants' attitudes towards the sexuality and sexual rights of the mentally handicapped.

The leader for this introductory session should be the trainer in charge, although an assistant can do the warming-up exercises, and lead a discussion if any introductory films are shown. A useful film to show parents and professionals is *On Being Sexual,* which presents various issues involving the sexuality of mentally handicapped persons. Another discussion-provoking film on the rights of this group is *Board and Care,* a moving, unrequited-love story of two Down's Syndrome adolescents.

Session II   Filling in the Gaps of Knowledge

Because so few people receive education about human sexuality, it is safe to assume that most participants will have only meagre knowledge about it. The trainees should be given as much factual knowledge as time allows. An expert on the subject of sexuality can be asked to lecture and answer questions. If the training period is too short to include a special presentation on the subject, the participants should be made aware of what they need to know, and motivated to use resources to secure this information on their own. Presenting participants with detailed information is important because they may need factual knowledge in order to teach or counsel the clients. It should stimulate them to pursue the subject further, and help them to examine their attitudes. The participants could be asked to read a textbook on sexuality prior to the training course to give them some idea of the scope of their knowledge, and prepare them for discussion during the course. The group could also be given a short test on the facts of sexuality. If the test is coded trainees correct their own tests, discussing their questions afterwards. Topics covered should include:

(1) male and female anatomy
(2) the facts of human reproduction
(3) the medical aspects of the sexuality of the mentally handicapped and how they differ from those not handicapped
(4) human sexual behaviour and human sexual response
(5) genetic counselling
(6) venereal disease
(7) masturbation
(8) body changes during puberty, menopause

Session III   Personal Examination of Attitudes towards Sexuality

As mentioned before, any training course that involves sexuality must focus on the attitudes and feelings of the individual participants. Goals here help people to:

(1) get in touch with their feelings about their own sexuality
(2) become more comfortable with them
(3) be able to accept and deal with others sexual behaviour.

Our experience has proved that merely using lectures, films, readings, or even informal discussions may not fully prepare some trainees for teaching or counselling; they need also to develop the ease derived from an active, sometimes painful, effort to overcome discomfort in discussing sexuality. In presenting this particular aspect the participants should become emotionally involved in the subject to the extent that they can recognize some of their own guilt, negative, and uncomfortable feelings. It is hoped they will be able to discard some of these troublesome attitudes when they recognise that many of them are formed by irrational forces or negative conditioning during early childhood.

With this in view, the participants should be involved in a self-confrontation process exposing them to emotional experiences that will force them to recognize feelings; and at the same time give them the opportunity to share these feelings with others. Various procedures can accomplish this; the method used will depend on the leadership, the group, and the resources available. If a trainer is not experienced in this area, it might be advisable to ask an expert in sexuality training to conduct such a session, sometimes titled an "SAR" (Sexual Attitude Reassessment). Since the subject matter will mainly focus on the participants, it may not be necessary for this resource person to be an expert in mental handicap.

During this process, factors that influence the attitudes of the participants should be considered, such as:

(1) the nature of their own sexual drives
(2) their past and present cultural or religious environments
(3) the process of personality development, such as the quality of understanding and tenderness experienced during their early childhood and their degree of satisfaction in their roles as male or female
(4) how they received their education about sex and

(5) some of the charged sexual experiences of traumatic nature that almost everyone has experienced at one time or another.

An excellent film to introduce this section is *Looking For Me,* which uses dance therapy to demonstrate the importance of being comfortable with one's own body and the expression of feelings through body movement.

A radical (but if used well, effective) method of attitudinal examination is the use of films that present explicit sexual activity performed by people of various types and ages, such as the Multi-Media or Focus Films. These films were produced primarily for training medical students, but are currently being more widely used for training other professionals in the U.S. Viewing these films usually causes the participants' feelings to surface—embarrassing or shaming some, shocking, disgusting, angering others. Some trainees will enjoy certain films and become "turned on". Forcing the participants' feelings out on a common ground is a challenging task never to be treated lightly; however, it can be effectively used to accomplish what is needed for this aspect of training. These films should always be followed by small group discussions, so that the trainees can express their feelings and attitudes and recognize their similarities to and differences from those of others. Usually trainees' thresholds of discomfort in discussing sex are lowered during the process and some of the undersirable attitudes held by some group members are eased by discussing them with the more flexible members.

If films are not available to aid in examining attitudes and establishing more comfort, other methods may be used, such as values clarification exercise, also using small group discussions. An important aspect of this method is asking the participants to talk about early sexual experiences and misconceptions held as children about sexuality (Morrison and Price 1974). For example; conjuring up early experiences of sexual experimentation and the results if caught can be fun and effective.

Whatever method that encourages the participants to think, feel, evaluate, and discuss should be successful. Resource people assisting in this session should be comfortable with their own sexuality and able to communicate easily about the subject with others. They also should be skilful in perceiving the feelings of other people and in helping them handle their emotions.

After attitudes about sexuality in general are examined and discussed by the group additional topics should be added, such as: What attitudes are held about the sexuality of the mentally handicapped? Do trainees honestly believe this special group shares a common sexual drive with the non-handicapped population? Will trainees objectively and comfortably accept the sexuality of their clients in dealing with their behaviour?

One of the most difficult areas participants encounter in the training experience is usually the discussion of masturbation. Yet discussion of this subject is one of the most important because masturbation may be the only sexual outlet possible for some mentally handicapped persons to enjoy. The myths surrounding masturbation must be dispelled and the differences between masturbation as desirable or undesirable explored. Most individuals have difficulty in expressing their deeper feelings, and especially their own masturbatory experiences. Some trainees can talk *ad infinitum* about most of their sexual experiences, but when it comes to masturbation they are greatly inhibited. It is not absolutely necessary for the participants to speak of their personal experiences with masturbation so long as they are conscious of their feelings and can deal comfortably and objectively with the sexual behaviour of others.

Session IV Issues in Socialization of the Mentally Handicapped

Topics dealing with various aspects of socialization programmes and interpersonal relationships of both sexes—friendships, dating, marriage, and parenting—should be included in the training. There are numerous special problems that confront the mentally handicapped in forming social relationships and many highly controverisal issues involving their intimate relationships with other people, marriage, and bearing children. Professionals find it increasingly important to include in their training programmes the social-sexual aspects of living. They are realizing that training for successful social living is as important for the mentally handicapped as providing them with academic and work skills. Thus professionals need preparation for being involved in socialization programmes and for counselling in social-sexual situations.

In an atmosphere of thoughtful discussion, goals for this session are:

(1) to give participants the opportunity to express feelings on the issues involved in heterosexual relationships, with sexual expression as a possible extension of these relationships

(2) to consider ways and means of establishing policies that will mean consistent treatment by staff involving sexual behaviour of their clients or students

(3) to introduce participants to strategies and to develop skills in counselling techniques in social-sexual related areas

(4) to inform participants of some socialization programmes currently offered and how they are implemented

(5) to inform participants about reports of the studies on marriage, parenthood, and the mentally handicapped

(6) to help trainees to examine aspects of marriage and parenthood from the viewpoints of parents, the mentally handicapped themselves, their prospective children, and the community.

Because homosexual behaviour has been a common occurrence especially among institutionalized, mentally handicapped people, the subject of homosexuality should be introduced. Discussion should include the definition of homosexuality and how it differs from homosexual behaviour. It is important for the participants to understand the difference between a temporary or superficial homosexual activity and the set homosexual patterns or lifestyle of a truly "gay" person. A description by a male and a female homosexual of how they become aware of their homosexuality and the problems they encounter can offer the trainees valuable insight into this subject. Problems that may exist in the homosexual behaviour of mentally handicapped people should be shared, with possible solutions offered.

Most participants are concerned about dealing with the handicapped in daily encounters between the sexes—holding hands, kissing, hugging, and (on very rare occasions when clients are discovered in hidden places) participating in more intimate sexual behaviour. Some professionals are delighted to see appropriate acts of affection and they regard these as signs of progress in the socialization process. Other professionals are obsessed with anxiety over affection between mentally handicapped individuals, causing them to be ill-at-ease in their attempts to channel sexual impulses into appropriate behaviour. Often staff members disagree with each other, and are too emotionally involved to solve social problems easily and wisely. The whole subject needs free and lengthy discussion, with participants offering their work experience as topics for discussion and for finding useful solutions to the problems of when, where, and how much freedom of sexual behaviour can be allowed.

Birth control methods, sterilization, and abortion should be presented by a combination of medical and family planning experts and professionals involved in counselling mentally handicapped adults who are sexually active. In the past mentally handicapped individuals were usually either sterilized or removed from society to prevent their reproducing. The picture did not change much with the advent of early contraceptives (diaphragm, foam, condom) since these contraceptives required some judgment and forethought for effective use—generally too much to expect from the mentally handicapped.

The latest methods of birth control (the pill, IUD, and injection) are much less dependent on judgment, thus offering possible alternatives to sterilization or virtual imprisonment to prevent mentally handicapped persons from reproducing. In addition, abortion is now legally available as a back-up procedure, should contraceptives fail. Sterilization is still a choice for when contraception is consistently ineffective. These alternative birth control methods offer greater dignity to mentally handicapped individuals and broaden their rights under the normalization principle. However, to arrive at the effective contraceptive method that is acceptable to them and that they are able to use can be a difficult task for the people responsible for this special group. Careful preparation of the individual handicapped woman for receiving birth control services and good follow-up counselling to reinforce motivation and education are mandatory for success. Focus this session on preparing participants for involvement in these tasks.

Session V   Sex Education for the Mentally Handicapped

The participants should learn to discuss the following:

I *Definitions*
A.   Sexuality can be defined as the integration of the biological, physiological, sociological, and psychological aspects of an

individual's personality which expresses his/her maleness or femaleness.

(1) Biological aspects refer to the existence of bodily parts and functions related to a specific gender

(2) Physiological aspects refer to the pleasure/pain that can be associated with any biological function.

(3) Sociological aspects refer to the impact of our sexuality upon our relationships with others in determining our life style.

(4) Psychological aspects refer to the impact of sexuality on self-image and feelings towards self.

B. Sex education can be defined as an instructional programme which addresses itself to the interaction of the sexually related biological, physiological, sociological, and psychological influences encountered from childhood through adulthood which determine sexual knowledge, values, and attitudes.

Sex education has three components:

(1) The learner
(2) The teacher
(3) the subject matter

C. The goal of sex education can be defined as the positive perception of the individual of his/her sexuality and its positive contribution towards the quality of life. For the mentally handicapped the special needs presented are to:

(1) Prevent victimization

(2) Prevent rejection by the community due to inappropriate socio-sexual behaviour

(3) Prevent need for experimentation which could result in potentially negative emotional and physical results

(4) Prevent further deterioration of self-image due to misinformation of body parts and functions

II. *Foundations of Sex Education*

A. Methods of learning

From birth people are continually educated in sexuality. As a result, most knowledge does not come from classroom instruction, but rather from one of the following methods encountered during a lifetime.

(1) Environmental—the kind of sex education absorbed from

the day we are born until the day we die. It is a conditioning process of which most people are unconscious.

(2) Experiential—the sex education taught informally on the spot, when the need or the question arises or when a particular situation lends itself to a teaching or counselling moment.

(3) Formal—sex education that is taught by a particular person, usually an instructor, to a selected group or individual, presented at a special time and place.

Thus everyone is both a teacher and a learner of sexuality. For parents and/or professionals, the role of significant adult to others creates an additional responsibility to be aware of the impact knowledge, attitudes, and values have on the environmental, experiential, or formal education of those influenced.

B. Qualities of a good sex educator

(1) Knows the basic subject matter

(2) Is knowledgable about the people being taught

(3) Is aware of specific characteristics of people which impair learning and uses methods and materials to increase the effectiveness of the teaching

(4) Comes to terms with his/her sexuality so that he/she need not struggle with unresolved conflicts, anxieties, and tensions

(5) Comes to terms with the language of sex, both technical and slang, and is able to use it and accept it freely from others

(6) Has accepted the beliefs that:
   (a) the goals of sex education are not to eliminate all sexual responses
   (b) sexual interest of behaviour is not sinful, intrinsically evil, or sick
   (c) need for controlling one's sexuality is not based on sex being intrinsically evil
   (d) sexual feelings need not give rise to guilt and self-deprecating feeling

(7) Is accepting and tolerant of the sexual behaviour, feelings and attitudes of others no matter how different their views

(8) Is imaginative, ingenious, and flexible when teaching, since the subject matter is difficult

(9) Has a sense of humour; sexuality should not be grim, although it is often treated as though it were

(10) Is honest and direct in manner of speech

(11) Is a person of emotional stability

(12) Believes in the right of all human beings to achieve their full potential

III. *Myths Surrounding Sex Education*
Some participants may need assurance that:
(1) Withholding information about sexuality from a person does deter him or her from participating in sex.
(2) Sex education does not stimulate or motivate students into sexual activity. Often, in fact, a clear understanding of sexual feelings will mean the ability to control them and may prevent grief for oneself and others.
(3) Sex education cannot be premature. If the material is too complicated or advanced for the child's understanding, it will be boring and the child will not listen. On the other hand, understanding a sexual phenomenon can come too late and can cause emotional upset and harm—for example, a girl's first sight of menstrual blood without understanding what it means and how to care for herself.

IV. *Meeting Specific Sex Educational Needs of the Mentally Handicapped*
The need and value of sex education for the mentally handicapped should be established along with a discussion of special considerations for these individuals, according to age and level of intelligence. Because methods of presenting sex education to the educable/ESN(M) and trainable handicapped/ESN(S) do differ, it is best to group the participants according to their specific interests and needs, such as:
Group 1. Sex-education techniques and curriculum for very young educable mentally handicapped children
Group 2. Sex-education techniques and curriculum for educable adolescents and adult mentally handicapped individuals
Group 3. Teaching appropriate social-sexual behaviour to very young trainable handicapped children
Group 4. Teaching appropriate social-sexual behaviour to adolescent and adult trainables

A. *Sex Education for the Educable Mentally Handicapped EMR's/ESN(M)*

The participants can be told that much of what can be given to the mildly or borderline mentally handicapped can be the same as that given to the normal population. However, the material should be presented more simply and concretely and with much repetition (the same method as is used in other education for them). If reading skills are limited, visual materials such as charts, pictures, movies, and models are essential.

Caution participants that whenever relationships are discussed— whether it be the meaning of being a friend or a sexual partner— responsibility and consideration for the other individual's values and possible emotional and social *consequences* should be emphasized. Discussions of sexual intercourse should include the fact that babies will be conceived as a result of sexual intercourse, unless definite precautions are taken. An attempt should be made to bring out the emotional and social consequences of whatever is discussed.

The students may or may not ask questions or discuss all topics freely; this will depend on their level of social communication and on the teacher's skills. It is imperative, however, to elicit what they already know, so that existing misinformation may be corrected. The same curriculum guides as those used for normal intellects may be used, as long as they are not regarded as goals that must be accomplished.

B. *Sex Education for the Trainable Mentally Handicapped TMR's/ ESN(S)*

Some of the special considerations to be discussed with participants in a training sesson for those who are interested in sex education for the trainable mentally handicapped are based on these assumptions:

(1) that this low intelligence group does not have a rational approach in expressing their sexuality
(2) that many of them do not direct their sexual feelings toward the opposite sex in an "organized" manner; and
(3) that much of their sexual behaviour may be auto-erotic.

This does not necessarily mean that they do not have sex drive or curiosity about sex. In fact, some of the difficulties these individuals have is because of their own clumsy attempts to satisfy their curiosity. (Course trainees may remember "playing doctor" games.)

Learning for the low level mentally handicapped is accomplished mainly experientially or visually, accompanied by the use of very short simple statements with simple pictures or hand demonstrations. Because most trainables cannot discuss facts rationally, the education process will be an acting out of a simple social situation in order to demonstrate what is appropriate socio-sexual behaviour in specific instances. For example, the group can act out how to greet strangers, friends, or loved ones properly. Most course participants have difficulty in planning sex education programme because of the wide range of abilities of their students. A circular diagram describing the levels of teaching usually helps considerably to clear up confusion of whom to teach what (see Figure 1).

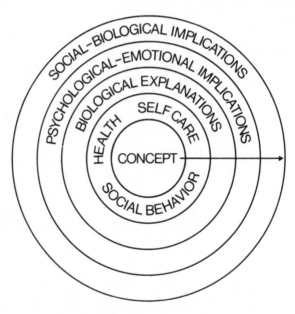

Figure 1: The Scarborough Method

The teacher should initiate the explanation at a level best understood by the students, where they may be expected to develop appropriate behavioural responses. This technique may be applied to many areas of human sexuality, always beginning with personal identity and self-care, and moving outward to embrace a broader scope of maleness or femaleness. When applicable, instruction may extend to more complex topics or issues dealing with social or psychological aspects (Kempton 1980).

C. *Curricula*

Discussion of the curricula should be kept to a minimum so the concept of flexibility is properly emphasised. However, participants should become familiar with at least one curriculum (see references and resources at the end of this chapter) prior to this session so they will be familiar with topics usually taught in sex-education programmes. In addition, they should know the main goals in teaching sex education to the mentally handicapped. Combining the two and utilizing the "Scarborough Method" will provide a basis on which to plan what to teach. The participants should be able to use their knowledge of the mentally handicapped to list the goals of sex education.

D. *Teaching Techniques*

The trainer should point out that there is no such thing as one ideal method of teaching. Each person and situation must be dealt with as an individual person and a specific situation. Therefore, no one programme can be suggested which will apply to all situations. Rather, if the opportunity to teach sexuality presents itself within the limitations of the job and existing policies, the following considerations should prove helpful:

(1) Before beginning be sure everyone (and if possible the student you will be working with) understands the disabilities and limitations that exist.

(2) Preview the student's record, or take the opportunity to evaluate what level of learning and moral development the person is capable of, and gauge what and how he/she can be taught.

(3) Find out what the person already knows first; draw out, don't pump in ideas.

(4) Start where the student is at his/her level of learning and moral development, as well as his/her emotional ability to handle the subject.

(5) Start where you are; if you don't feel comfortable in discussing some subjects, begin with those you do or refer to someone who is.

(6) Use the language or terminology of sexuality familiar to the person; use his words not yours. When appropriate, teach acceptable words.

69

(7) Keep explanations simple, honest, and direct.

(8) Don't wait for questions; the student may be too shy or not know what to ask.

(9) If the student shows immaturity by laughing or giggling, remind him/her of the seriousness of the matter; but also remember that it could be a release of tension and embarrassment, therefore to be allowed within reason.

(10) Keeping males and females together is appropriate in most cases. Exceptions should be based on certain subject matter or the needs of the individual learner.

(11) Don't lecture or moralize. Too much guilt is already associated with sex. Do emphasize, however, that sex is something private and mature with specific responsibilities.

(12) Whenever possible, use concrete, tangible, visual materials (see list at the end of this chapter).

(13) Use dramatic play whenever possible. There are three types of dramatic play that teachers of special education can use:

(a) *Pantomime* is "action without words," which is expressing feelings and thoughts through the use of the body without speech. Pantomime is the simplest form of dramatic play and is helpful for practicing and identifying actions and behaviour which do not involve dialogue. It is most effectively used with the non-verbal, the very young, or students with severe learning impairment.

(b) *Improvisation*—a scene which is planned in advance (who, where) but action and dialogue are left to the players. Observing students enact a scene in which they determine the outcome can be an excellent base for class discussion and can give a teacher insight into the ability of the students to make wise decisions. It is used most effectively with the moderately and mildly retarded, although all ages and most levels can learn from it.

(c) *Role Playing*—part of socio-drama in which a life problem is acted out. By changing roles, the individual is given an opportunity to find alternatives through various life situations. After the scene is enacted as directed, the students gain insight first by evaluating their feelings during the drama and, secondly, by evaluating the audience reaction to the presentation. This exercise is usually most effective with individuals who are able to communicate and interact.

Dramatic play has many benefits in addition to the insights the students will gain.

—It helps teach self-control
—It promotes a better self-image because it permits each student to receive praise for his or her strength and to improve performance
—It allows opportunities for interaction with classmates and teacher
—It helps the special student to distinguish between reality and unreality or, in simpler terms, pretend and real
—It is a very effective tool for teaching responsibility
—It can be used to reinforce socially acceptable behaviour and explore the possible consequences of such things as unwanted pregnancies, marriage, and parenthood (Kempton 1980).

The scope and application of role playing as an educational tool are determined by the imagination and enthusiasm of the teacher and the limitations of the students. Most impediments can be overcome with patience and hard work. The results will more than justify the effort.

Session VI   Working with Parents

During most training courses the constant question from the group is "What shall we do about the parents of the clients? They are so anxious, and many of them are restrictive about their children's sexuality. How do we deal with this?"

It is true that in some situations parents have inhibited the efforts of professionals to counsel or educate their children about sexuality, and differences between the professionals' and the parents' attitudes and methods of dealing with sexual behaviour can cause complications. Parents and professionals need each other in these days when confusion and controversy surround sex education. They do, in fact, have complementary roles, and the more they work together, the greater and faster will be the children's progress. Sex education should, and essentially does, lie with the parents. Whether they recognize it or not, they are constantly giving their children sex education. Silence in answer to a question is sex education. However, it is unlikely that parents will take the initiative in preparing themselves to meet all the special needs of their handicapped children in this area. Thus it falls to the professionals to lead the way by preparing themselves with the information and training necessary to teach effectively and to help when needed (Kempton 1975). Understanding parental attitudes and aptitudes is very important when it comes to making professional help acceptable. Therefore, any training course for professionals should equip the participants with information, understanding, and skills enabling them to help parents deal with the sexuality of their mentally handicapped children.

A. *The Main Goals of Session are:*

(1) To discuss and outline the dynamics of professionals and parents working together effectively
(2) To prepare the professional to give reassurance, support, and direction to parents, especially in dealing with the sexuality of their mentally handicapped children
(3) To allay participants' anxieties about parental criticisms
(4) To point out the role of the professional in sex education and the fact that, in some circumstances, he or she can accomplish more than the parent because of the social environment and teaching resources available to him or her
(5) To make participants aware of the fact that the professional can and should learn from the wise parent who is reality-oriented
(6) To help participants develop the skills to reach parents and the special techniques to handle the difficult subject matter of sexuality
(7) To prepare participants for special complications such as parents with negative attitudes, lack of acceptance by the community, and specific problems.

B. Since parents are to be the special topic at this session, we recommend that they be invited to attend or be represented. Here are some suggestions:

(1) Ask three or four parents to give a panel presentation describing their experiences, feelings, and concerns with regard to the sexuality of their children. (Participants should be reminded that these will be highly personalized viewpoints and should not be taken as established factual material or overall opinions.)

(2) Ask any expert who is experienced in working with parents to give a presentation; then ask a panel of parents to react.

(3) Show a film that is directed particularly to parents; ask a panel of parents to respond to it or lead a general discussion. The film *On Being Sexual* is recommended as it depicts a workshop on sexuality for parents of mentally handicapped children.

(4) Ask parents to join the training group and to participate informally in the general discussion of the session.

(5) Ask one or more siblings of a mentally handicapped individual to discuss with the group their experiences and feelings while growing up with a mentally handicapped brother or sister.

The following questions and answers have frequently been posed by parents of mentally handicapped children. We recommend that you deal with as many of these topics as possible during the session:

(1) How can I go about having my son/daughter sterilized?

(2) What shall I tell my son/daughter about sex?

(3) Will sex education cause him/her to experiment?

(4) Will sex education sexually stimulate my child?

(5) How can I prepare my daughter for menstruation?

(6) Our son/daughter tries to masturbate but doen't know how to reach a climax. What shall we do?

(7) How can we protect our daughter from being sexually used?

Participants may also be given the opportunity to role play situations with parents. They should be given some guidelines on how to organize meetings with parents to discuss sexuality and how to conduct counselling sessions with them. A training course outline for parents should be offered to the group in the event that they could conduct one. However, participants should be forewarned that finding parents who are willing to devote their time and to become closely involved in a training course is unlikely. A training course sample is outlined on page 89 in the training guide (Kempton and Forman 1980).

Session VII The Organization of Sex Education and Sex Counselling Programmes and the Politics of Sex

The trainees probably will ask for practical suggestions on how to use their training experience in their own settings; therefore, a discussion should be held on setting up various types of programmes and the politics involved. If possible, individuals who have already planned and implemented programmes should act as resource people. One recommended strategy: participants now graduates of the training course make a quiet survey of the attitudes that their collegues and administrative staff generally hold towards sex education and counselling. What are their attitudes about the sexuality of the mentally handicapped? Those who will support staff training and sex education programmes should be identified. If the graduate feels some resistance it may be wise to document examples of clients who have had special problems because of lack of knowledge about sex or training for appropriate sexual behaviour. It may also be advisable to analyze the community attitudes about socialization programmes that already exist. A committee can be organized to pool ideas and add support to the project. It is wise to establish priorities for activities that predictably will meet with the least amount of resistance. The more complicated and controversial issues may be postponed until the climate is favourable.

The financial situation should be examined: how much support may be secured for resources and training? Admittedly, one can plan more freely if special funds are available but action should not be delayed because of a lack of funds.

A very important task of every agency or institution is to develop a set of policies on how to deal with sexual behaviour and the kind of sex education programmes it wants. These policies should include what the institution, agency, or school regard as the social-sexual rights of their mentally handicapped clients. It is very difficult in any setting where sex education or counselling programmes are being instituted to make any progress unless these policy statements are written, as they will be the base line for consistency in teaching and counselling the mentally handicapped. Unresolved problems and unstated procedures may often be inhibiting factors for some staff or a constant source of tension between them and the administrators.

The procedures of policy-making vary, but in many settings a committee does the work. Ideally, this group should consist of members who would be a cross section of all the professions represented in that setting. The committee drafts the policies and then presents them to the administrator for approval. (See Chapter 4 for more details on policy making.)

Summary

The training described in this chapter is a model that has emerged from presenting hundreds of training courses, a model that is meant to be used flexibly. It is highly recommended that the trainers use many variations, both in programme context and style of presentation, to adjust to the various situations encountered from place to place. The number of hours allocated for the training course will determine how much detail can be presented, how many subjects can be dealt with, as well as how much time can be used for group intereaction. Obviously the longer the course usually the better the results, although this is not always true. One of the most important determinants of success is the perceptive ability of the trainer to size up the group and rearrange the programme according to its make-up, eliminating or adding as needed. In certain parts of the US and in some countries, such as Singapore and Sri Lanka, showing film of explicit sexual activity would cause such a furore that all else in the course could be ineffective. In other parts of the United States and Canada these films seem to be the best way to urge people to admit discomfort or come to grips with their attitudes. The level of knowledge varies both from individual to individual and from group to group. The trainer must be prepared to retreat or advance in presenting factual information. The discussion policy, issues, and morality should be relevant to the needs of the group as well as the laws and mores of the community from which the participants come. These and many other variables must be taken into consideration.

It is a difficult task for the trainers to meet all the needs of all the group members, especially if there are more than 20 participants. At times small group discussions or role playing are necessary in order to give participants the opportunity to air their feelings and opinions. There should be a group facilitator for every 9 to 12 participants. These leaders are especially needed for helping the trainer understand both the moods and the needs of the participants, as well as for implementing an effective interaction process.

Training courses in sexuality are interesting, challenging, and can be greatly satisfying. Adding the dimension of helping to assure the social-sexual rights of mentally handicapped persons through training professionals to implement these rights gives even more depth and purpose to the goals trainers hope to achieve.

REFERENCES

Kempton, W. (1975). Sex Education—a co-operative effort of parent and teacher. *Exceptional Children* 41, 8, 531–35.

Kempton, W. (1980). *Sex Education for Persons with Disabilities that Hinder Learning.* Philadelphia: Planned Parenthood of Southeastern Pennsylvania (2nd edition). ⋅

Kempton, W. and Forman, R. (1980). *Guidelines for Training in Sexuality and the Mentally Handicapped.* Philadelphia: Planned Parenthood of Southeastern Pennsylvania (2nd edition).

Morrison, E. and Price, M. (1974). *Values in Sexuality.* New York: Hart Publishing Co. Inc.

RESOURCES*

Teaching and Training Materials for Parents and Professionals

On Being Sexual, a film featuring Sol Gordon and Winifred Kempton in discussions with young adults and parents. Accompanied by a discussion guide by Jeff Bassin and Teel Ackerman and a training package for workshop leaders. Available from Stanfield House, 900 Euclid Ave., Box 3208, Santa Monica, CA 90403.

Human Sexuality and the Mentally Retarded, a filmstrip for parents, teachers and institutional staff regarding providing sexuality information to the retarded. Available from Planned Parenthood of Southeastern Pennsylvania, 1220 Sansom Street, Philadelphia, PA 19107.

The ABC of Sex Education for Trainable Persons, a film designed for in-service training in institutions which can also be used by parents for at-home instruction. Available from Hallmark Films, 51 New Plant Court, Owens Mills, MD 21117.

The How and What of Sex Education for Educable Persons, training film for educators and parents. Available from Hallmark Films, 51 New Plant Court, Owens Mills, MD 21117.

Fertility Regulation for the Mentally Handicapped, a training film for parents and educators. Available from Hallmark Films, 51 New Plant Court, Owens Mills, MD 21117.

Feeling Good About Yourself, a film/videotape demonstrating the teaching of socialization skills to the mentally handicapped. Parennial Education, Inc., 477 Roger Williams, P.O. Box 855 Ravinia, Highlands Park, IL 60035.

Looking For Me, a dance therapist demonstrates the importance of body movement. Available from Multi-Media Resource Center, 1525 Franklin St., San Francisco, CA 94019.

Board and Care, a moving film depicting the "love story" of two Down's Syndrome youths and their parents reactions to their social development. Could be useful for stimulating discussions with a group of mentally handicapped persons and/or parents. Available from Pyramid Films, 1537 14th St., Box 1048, Santa Monica, CA 90406.

Focus Films, New York City, N.Y.

Multimedia Films, San Francisco, CA.

---

*For resources available in Britain see Chapter 8, and Craft, A. (1980). *Health Hygiene and Sex Education for Mentally Handicapped Children, Adolescents and Adults: A review of audio-visual resources.* Health Education Council

Materials for Teaching and Testing the Mentally Handicapped

Sexuality and the Mentally Handicapped, by Winifred Kempton. A nine part slide series dealing with all aspects of human sexuality, with accompanying teacher's guide. Available from Stanfield Film Associates. Box 851, Pasadena, CA 91102.

Socio-Sexual Knowledge and Attitudes Test (SSKAT), designed for the developmentally disabled. Available from Stoelting Co, Chicago, IL. Test developed by Joel Wish, K. McCombs, and B. Edmonson.

Human Sexuality: A Portfolio for the Mentally Retarded, ten separate drawings on stiffened paper, with discussion suggestions printed on the back of each plate for the teacher. Available from Planned Parenthood of Seattle-King County, 2211 E. Madison Ave., Seattle, WA 98112.

EASE: An Empirically Validated Sex Education Curriculum for the Mentally Handicapped. Keyed for use with slide series cited above. Published by Stanfield Film Associates, Box 851, Pasadena, CA 91102.

Effie Dolls, visual aid mannequins, handmade rag-doll creations designed to aid in explanation of human anatomy. Male doll is complete with genitals. Female doll is pregnant. Available from Mrs. Judith Franing, 4812 48th Ave., Moline, IL 61625.

Jim Jackson Models of Human Genital Anatomy—life size, life-like, exact reproductions of male and female sexual organs. Includes uterus and tubes, erect penis, and vasectomy. Can be used for training professionals and educating mentally handicapped persons. Available from Jim Jackson, 16 Laurel Street, Arlington, Mass. 02174.

CHAPTER 4

Counselling Parents and Care Staff on the Sexual Needs of Mentally Handicapped People

Winifred Kempton and Frank Caparulo

All mentally handicapped persons are sexual beings. While many may not enter into active sexual relationships with partners, or marry, or procreate, they are sexual. This implies that they experience sexual drives and behaviours; they may masturbate for sexual release, become attracted to and be intimate with someone, and have a fantasy life. How well parents and care staff understand and deal with these normal sexual activities will determine to a great extent how much sexual freedom the mentally handicapped population is to enjoy.

In this chapter we will discuss how parents and care staff: (1) envision the sexuality and sexual expression of the mentally handicapped as normal; (2) may view both without anxiety and/or revulsion; and (3) accept this part of the personhood with dignity.

Sexuality is a delicate issue to broach with both mentally retarded clients and their parents. Reasons for counselling should be clear and succinct. In order to make the client's life more fulfilling the counsellor may assist the client in resolving any home problems or barriers that interfere with the attainment of adulthood, and in gaining as much independence as possible and/or in expressing his or her sexuality in a wholesome and appropriate fashion. The counsellor should be prepared to offer couples counselling for those in relationships, premarital counselling for those who request it, marriage counselling for those who need it, and sex counselling when it is possible.

Attitudes Toward the Sexuality of Mentally Handicapped Persons

However before we can specifically deal with counselling issues for parents and care givers we should consider some of the barriers they erect, consciously and unconsciously, which hinder their ability to cope with the sexual behaviour and sexual growth of mentally handicapped persons. Such obstructions are built on various attitudes and beliefs which need to be questioned and examined.

In their book *Sex Education and Counselling of Special Groups* Warren Johnson and Winifred Kempton describe four sequential stages of attitudes relevant to the sexuality and sexual expressions of the mentally handicapped: (1) to eliminate their sexuality, (2) to tolerate their sexuality, (3) to accept their sexuality, and (4) to cultivate their sexuality (Johnson and Kempton, 1981). As the titles of these philosophies are almost self explanatory, our descriptions will be brief.

(1) *Eliminate the Sexuality of the Mentally Handicapped*

Many who profess this attitude (or philosophy) believe generally that sexual expression should be limited to marriage and engaged in only by those who function as intellectually "normal". This philosophy holds that: (a) masturbation is sinful; (b) other sexual expression or stimulation is bad; (c) the mentally handicapped don't experience the same drives and needs as do the non-handicapped population; and (d) sterilization is the best way to handle the potential sexuality of the mentally handicapped. Physical restraints (e.g., tying hands, corporal punishment) and medical procedures (e.g., castration, total hysterectomies) have been resorted to as a means of eliminating the sexual expression of mentally handicapped persons, and of late, there have been experiments with drugs to mitigate the libido.

Knowing what we do about the emotional needs of the mentally handicapped, we view believers in the theory of elimination as medieval in thought. *How* the mentally handicapped express their sexuality is our legitimate concern; whether or not they should be allowed to express it, is not.

(2) *Tolerate the Sexuality of the Mentally Handicapped*

Persons holding this view agree that the mentally handicapped are sexually normal, or nearly so. Understandably, the majority of parents take this position. They may have read and thought about the problem but are not convinced that mentally handicapped

79

persons can handle the responsibilities that accompany sexual expression. They are concerned that such expression by those labelled atypical will cause problems; so because of societal prejudices (Caparulo and Caparulo, 1979) they are unable to allow their offspring to develop psychosexually as normally as possible.

People who hold a philosophy of toleration seem to measure the quality of relationships by the parameters they set ideally for their own lives but which are often unrealistic for special groups. The literature on marriage and the mentally handicapped demonstrates the error in this thinking (Mattinson 1973; Hall 1974; Bass 1979; and Craft and Craft 1979). Many mentally handicapped couples marry for companionship and to escape loneliness. Who is to judge whether or not theirs are quality relationships; each relationship should be judged individually for its quality: generalizations are difficult to make. Should love, romantic love, be the only prerequisite for marriage between handicapped people? Western society continues to regard romantic love as the basis for most marital relationships, despite the rising divorce rate.

(3) *Accept their Sexuality*

We advocate this attitude for several reasons; (a) by United Nations decree and by moral law the mentally handicapped have the same rights as anyone else, including the right to be sexual and to express it in appropriate fashion; (b) there is little chance of protecting the handicapped from exposure to undesirable "sex education" gleaned from R and X rated films, television, magazines, and pornography; (c) to accept the sexuality and sex expression of mentally handicapped persons indicates that we believe they have normal emotional needs to love and be loved, to show affection, to establish relationships, and to express their sexuality in a healthy manner. We recognize that acceptance of these needs is not easy for all parents and care-givers to develop; while they may recognize the need for change, they anxiously hold back, a process that we need to help them through at their own pace.

(4) *Cultivate their Sexuality*

This philosophy can be generally practiced if society permits it, if parents feel comfortable with it, and care-givers can deal with it. With this attitude the mentally handicapped can be encouraged and helped to enrich their lives through sexual expression which can be accomplished through humane policies and programmes, training for parents and staff, sex education and training for clients, and supportive sex counselling.

This school of thought is not readily or widely accepted and seldom seriously considered but it offers a basis for a progressive policy that can be translated into healthy living practices.

Counselling Parents

It is important to note that today's parents are products of the sexual values prevalent a generation or more ago. Hence they may need sex education and counselling to assist them in dealing with today's sexual perspectives and their children's reactions.

Parents present a variety of expressions in response to the first signs of secondary sex characteristics and sexual behaviour in their mentally handicapped children. Fear and anxiety are often aroused, especially by a female child's physical development such as the first menses (menarche), an occurance that arouses anxiety about the potential for pregnancy.

Not all responses from parents are such that counselling is indicated. Some parents respond positively: "Our children are as entitled as anyone to a natural sex life. They have the same needs for physical release and emotional closeness. If they meet someone they can love, who returns that love, they should marry and be given whatever support is necessary to make the marriage work." These parents usually add: "The question of their bearing children requires serious thought and planning."

Goodman (1973 and 1975) presents us with an assortment of other parental responses that require some type of counselling and/or education. Views commonly found are: (1) denial of the sexuality of their children; (2) a pseudo-enlightened attitude towards sexuality; (3) confused and ambivalent thinking; (4) a strict moralistic attitude; and (5) an over-protective "eternal child" attitude towards their handicapped offspring.

1. *Denial of Sexuality or the "Pandora's Box Complex"*

Parents who deny their children's sexuality are usually frightened and uninformed. In most cases they have attempted to rear their offspring as asexual, not out of malice but out of fear that, "because of the handicap he/she will not be able to handle all the complexities that go along with sex." Thus sex may never be mentioned because it would unleash uncontrollable urges (the "Pandora's Box" complex); it's better to keep them innocent and as eternal children (Caparulo and Caparulo, 1979). In such cases the counsellor must move slowly to relieve parental fears and anxieties as they arise. Parents need to be helped to understand that sexuality does not necessarily connote sexual intercourse, that expressing one's sexuality is more likely to involve understanding and enjoying one's body and gender role. Parents can also be reassured by seeing that most mentally handicapped persons prefer traditional and stereotypic roles, because such roles are structured, accepted, more clearly defined, and thus easier to understand.

2. *Pseudo-enlightened Attitudes*

Parents who deny their children's sexuality are like those with pseudo-enlightened attitudes, professing a restrictive definition of sexuality. These restrictions deter healthy socio-sexual development or close interaction with others. This group is against marriage, adopting the self-fulfilling prophesy, "Marriage is hard enough for me; there is no way that my daughter can be successful as a wife, so we don't encourage boy/girl relationships."

Such parents measure all heterosexual relationships by their own experiences of marriage. They don't see how two mentally handicapped persons can have a successful marriage. Again, as we have said before, the quality of a relationship between a female and a male may not require all of the emotional investment envisioned by parents. We need to remind parents that denying their handicapped children the "normal" model of dating and marriage reinforces the concept that they are not "normal", that something is wrong with them.

Parents with these attitudes look within themselves to find answers; they may need guidance to resolve what is "good" for their offspring and education to strengthen their positive feelings.

3. *Confused or Ambivalant Attitude about Sexuality*

In this group are parents who give non-verbal permission (perhaps for self-satisfaction) for behaviours that are inappropriate in public. When the mentally handicapped offspring acts as he has been allowed to at home, he is punished by the very person who has subtly granted permission for such behaviour. This can be, and is, very confusing to the youngster; he may test his home behaviour in another setting, i.e., the sheltered workshop, school, or at a social event. Then when the sexual behaviour is reported to the parent, panic results, and we hear "I don't know where he/she learned it."

In such a situation the counsellor needs to determine what is occurring in the home to demonstrate to the parents without blaming them, the part they have played. These parents need to be made more aware of the human needs of their offspring, how their children's behaviour affects others, and their own roles as primary adult models.

4. *Moralistic Attitude*

As Hall (1975) states, "This response envisions sex as permissible only in marriage and primarily for the purpose of procreation. This response, coupled with the belief that the retarded person is not capable of accepting marital responsibilities, is one of the most difficult to deal with; any expression of sexuality is viewed with alarm."

Parents who display these attitudes should be treated with caution. It is important that the counsellor show an appreciation of the parents' position on this issue. Strategies for intervention must be well thought out; progress is usually slow. The parents' viewpoint represents lifetime learning and deserves respect for its values, beliefs and wishes. If parents feel pressured to change and threatened by differing values they may withdraw their child from counselling and keep him or her at home where they have total control which is better than taking a step backwards, at least.

5. *Over-protective Attitude: "Sex is too Risky"*

Perske (1972) remarks that this parental attitude "endangers the retarded person's human dignity and tends to keep him or her from experiencing the normal taking of risks in life, which are necessary for human growth and development."

This situation could be caused by the lack of knowledge of their offsprings' needs, their own inability to risk untried experiences, the eternal child syndrome, or other reasons. The counsellor's task is to help resolve these conflicts as much as possible.

Parents who exhibit any one or more of the five views discussed above (denial of sexuality, pseudo-enlightened or moralistic attitude, double-standard sexuality or over-protection) may be helped. The counsellor should be as non-judgemental as possible in approach; respect the parents' values and beliefs; and assure them that the quality of their child's life is the ultimate goal. One of the most important tasks throughout the process is to provide education to correct any myths and misconceptions surrounding sexuality and sexual expressions.

In the book *Sexual Counseling of Special Groups* Warren Johnson explains a clinic approach to the sex education and counselling of parents about the sexuality of their children, that he has found efficient and reasonable effective:

1. *The parents receive basic classroom instruction on topics which past experience has demonstrated to be of greatest common interest.* Perhaps only five or six topics are dealt with because of time limitations (about 30 minutes). But these are intended to serve as a model for informed, objective confrontation with an analysis of other subjects as well. The underlying theme of the presentation can be stated in the following terms: Since most common sexual and sex-related behaviors are in in themselves harmless or, perhaps, even beneficial, why make needless problems of them?

2. *A challenge is presented as follows:* It used to be the responsibility of the parent or professional person to eliminate sexual expression among most special group members, as among children. Today, however, there is not just one possibility, there are three: (a) still try to eliminate sexual expression; (b) to tolerate or even accommodate it; or (c) to cultivate it as one might cultivate other personality resources such as intelligence, artistic ability or sports aptitude. Which, I ask parents, is your choice? Most seem willing to accept the challenge and try to think out just where they stand. Certainly there has been a shift to choice (b); but a few people opt for (c).

3. *Questions are then invited.* The gathering begins as instruction and ends in effect as small group counseling and then individual counseling. Parents always bring up sex-related problems of their children at this point. Pedagogy shifts to counseling, with other parents spontaneously becoming involved as they have experiences to recount, questions to raise, solutions to propose. If the person who posed the problem does not seem to be applying information presented earlier, others call this to his attention. Sometimes, within minutes, there are fascinating changes in outlook and reassessment of situations. Factual misconceptions and moral confusions often quickly disappear as people begin to deal objectiverly with facts, specific situations and the possible meanings of behavior. Parents who do not have the time or inclination to bring up

problems in the group come forward for a few minutes of counseling at the end.

Over the years, I have been impressed by the response of these parents. There have been hundreds of them now, and they represent something of a cross-section of our society, socio-economically and educationally. Even in the early years, only occasionally did a parent become upset by my bluntly presented information and discussion which unavoidably often set traditional views topsy-turvy. My distinct impression is that professionals have been underestimating the public. School administrators, teachers, physicians and politicians tend to feel the need to protect the public from the realities of sex. (Johnson and Kempton, 1981.)

One counselling technique often helpful is to get parents to assess their attitudes on sexual issues. This could be accomplished by asking them to rank some sexual topics, from the most threatening to the least threatening to deal with. When both parents are involved, they should do the ranking independently of each other; this may reveal which parent is easier for the counsellor to work with. Items suggested for the assessment: sexual behaviour, sex education, menstruation, care and cleanliness of the body, masturbation, dating, sexual intercourse outside of marriage, marriage, venereal disease, birth control, homosexuality, procreation. This assignment should be followed by a non-judgmental discussion of the parents' fears and anxieties.

Care Staff Involvement in the Social-Sexual Development of Clients

Until recently in America, when new staff members were hired at an institution for the mentally handicapped they would not be told that part of their duties would be to handle the client's sexuality or sexual expressions. The social-sexual development of the clients should be a concern of the direct care staff, for unless an initial commitment is made to this aspect of their responsibilities, people who are mentally handicapped will not realize their full potential. When hired, staff at all levels should be made aware of their responsibilities, according to the policies of the institution. Orientation or training should be made available which would include dealing with the social, emotional, psychological and sexual needs of the clients. (A training course is described in this text by Winifred Kempton, see Chapter 3.)

To ensure participation of staff, there must also be a commitment from the administration to staff's input in the development of policies that will provide structure and support. Participation could mean a temporary task force or a permanent "sexuality" or "socialization" committee.

Suggested Task Force Model

The initial step, after bringing the task force members together, is to develop its goals and objectives and to identify "resource" people who are interested, motivated, and dedicated enough to the cause of sexual rights to contribute time and energy. These persons should then be organized into a working committee. This group would:

(1) Create guidelines with administrative support that will provide consistency in dealing with the sexuality and sexual expressions of the mentally handicapped.

(2) Provide training courses for staff according to their needs. For example, in the United States the state of Connecticut organized such a task force and then divided into subcommittees that represented major issues that needed to be investigated. Each subcommittee approached its topic through in-depth research, consultation, and discussion. The subcommittees of this Connecticut model were:

A. Mental and Physical Health Committee

This group examined the physiological, psychological, and emotional aspects of sexuality and the mentally handicapped. Topics covered were: reproduction, genetic implications, sexuality and the multihandicapped (physical and mental), venereal diseases and their control, gynecological examinations and concerns, contraception, and sterilization.

B. Legal Committee

This group researched and reviewed local and national laws related to sexuality control, and sterilization. It also incorporated the recommendations of national groups and agencies involved with the mentally handicapped. The committee prepared the task force recommendations for possible legislative action. Other legal concepts that were explored and needed special interpretations were "informed consent" and "competency".

C. *Resource Committee*

This group's task was to: (1) identify and evaluate resource personnel (staff, school teachers, and physicians, etc.) within the geographic area of the institution; (2) review curricula, audiovisual materials, teacher guides, and training courses; (3) identify the needs and existing gaps in services and materials; (4) recommend staff training courses available in the community.

D. *Philosophy Committee*

This group investigated and shared ideologies with other agencies and institutions. It investigated the underlying values and morality of the project and then developed the philosophy for the task force. This committee was representative of specific community and professional groups as well as institution personnel. It co-ordinated the activities of all the subcommittees to ensure the development of common goals, maintained effective communications, and eliminated duplication of efforts.

E. *Implementation Committee*

This group was responsible for the compilation, dissemination, and implementation of the total report of the task force. This was done after the report was accepted by the appropriate governing boards including the governor's committee.

F. *Human Sexuality Committee*

After the final report was adopted, representatives of each subcommittee formed a human sexuality committee at their thirteen respective settings (eleven regional centres and two training schools). The responsibilities of this committee included: (1) training staff, (2) implementating policies, (3) recommending curricula, (4) developing and reviewing audiovisual materials, and (5) helping make decisions on resolving problems not addressed by the policy.

*A Suggested Policy Statement**

The mandate of [the residential unit or facility] is to provide and promote services that enhance the development and normalization

*Adopted from: Policy on Sexuality 17, Department of Mental Retardation, State of Connecticut, U.S.A.

of the institution's clients. An important part of personal development is growth as a sexual being. Hence, the institution has a responsibility to address and deal with sexuality and sexual expression. With that responsibility comes the necessity to provide sexual education and counselling based on the developmental levels and chronological ages of the individuals served, and consistent with cultural norms.

This mission has as its ideal to provide dignified treatment for the development of the client's fullest potential with respect for their personal dignity and right to privacy, consistent with individualized treatment plans.

In essence, the institution's policy is based on the premises that everyone is born a sexual being and that sexuality is a common bond with the nonhandicapped. Differences do occur in the ways and methods of fulfilment that individuals use. The handicapped have the right to choose among the same alternatives available to other people for their sexual and emotional expressions. Education: the institution will offer sexual education and sex counselling not limited to but including emotional, spiritual, biological, responsible, appropriate, inappropriate and decision-making aspects of an individual's sexual behaviour and protection against exploitation and abuse. The education and counselling programmes should stress that sexuality is what people *are,* not something they *do.* It is a continuum of learning about men and women. It will include the levels of understanding and responsibility appropriate to each person.

Staff need to help the client achieve his/her desires, consistent with cultural norms. Succinctly stated, it is the policy of the institution:

—that sexual education, sex counselling, and the client's sexuality are valid, important issues and concerns.
—that institution staff must respond to client's questions, concerns, and actions with sensitivity and dignity, in a relaxed, mature, professional manner corresponding to the client's abiities to comprehend.
—that institute staff must support and protect the mentally handicapped person's rights of self expression of sexuality and with respect for other clients' rights
—that all sexual education and sex counselling should be appropriate for the client's age group, and/or functioning level

—that a Human Sexuality Committee representing all staff levels should be formed to deal with and make final decisions on cases and incidents involving sexual expressions that need resolution. This committee should be responsible for overseeing staff training, client training and education, policy implementation, and curriculum decisions.

There are other models that can be followed. In some settings much of the work is done by only a few individuals. Whatever model is used is unimportant, as long as a structure of consistent methods of treatment for residents is established to be utilized by the care staff.

Sex Counsellors for Mentally Handicapped Persons

Problems and Qualifications

There is a scarcity of persons who are able to adequately counsel mentally handicapped persons about their sexuality. An examination of some of the facts may lead to corrective action and widen the number of available qualified counsellors.

1. The necessity for sex counselling for the mentally handicapped has not been honestly faced because, historically, society has believed this group to be asexual. Care-givers in the past have refused to deal with clients' sexuality and sexual expressions except in a punitive manner, aiming mainly to eradicate sexuality and thus reinforcing the asexual theme. Fortunately, today professionals on all levels are admitting that many serious problems they face are sex-related.

2. There is a paucity of hard data and literature on how to counsel the mentally handicapped. Even with growing awareness of the problem, a person searching for a training course in human sexuality or sex counselling for the mentally handicapped is hard pressed to find one. Those who do train sex counsellors frequently have to recommend trial and error methods in dealing with a problem.

3. Techniques used for the general population are often not applicable to the mentally handicapped. Since they have been reared as asexual they have been sexually abused and exploited, and function at a low level of intelligence. This group presents a multitude of problems unfamiliar to most professionals. Most mentally handicapped persons are characteristically unable to deal

with abstractions so everything must be presented in concrete, visual form and or in the form of experience as in role play, feedback or rehearsal.

4. Many aspects of sexual counselling involve highly controversial issues. Professionals and parents may have diverse values and beliefs on dating, birth control, marriage, parenthood, and various methods of sexual expression for mentally handicapped persons. The spectrum of these opinions may range from no sexual rights to all the sexual rights enjoyed by the "normal" population.

5. Sex education and sex counselling with the mentally handicapped are often synonymous. Because of their meagre knowledge of all aspects of sexuality it is usually necessary to give them basic information before the counsellor can expect to guide or change the behaviour of clients. For example, it is not unusual for a family planning counsellor to have a mentally handicapped person or couple present themselves for contraceptive counselling who have no knowledge of sexual intercourse or basic sexual anatomy and physiology. It is obvious that teaching must precede counselling in these situations.

6. Positive or negative sex counselling depends on the ability of the sex counsellor to separate his/her own attitudes, values and beliefs from what are the perceived needs of the clients.

7. Because there are too few counsellors, it is often necessary for care staff to assume that role because: (1) there may be no "expert" available, (2) sex counselling necessitates a trusting relationship which many care staff have established, (3) the strategic time to counsel is on the spot, when questions are asked and behaviours occur (Kempton, 1975a), and (4) if a situation is not dealt with immediately the opportunity to help may never come along again.

8. Complications may arise if the client is multihandicapped. Fifty per cent of all spastics (cerebral palsied) are mentally handicapped (Cruickshank, 1966). Strategies must suit the handicap and its limitations; such as blindness, deafness, or retardation.

9. Staff of institutions are often confined by restrictions imposed by administrators or parents. This is especially so where humane policies and guidelines do not exist. If policies and guidelines do exist certain precautions should be taken. Sessions should be audio-taped, after obtaining consent; while counselling an unstable or acting-out client the door of the room should be left open and a

colleague should be able to see both client and counsellor at all times; if the client is a minor, parents should be involved.

What constitutes the need for sexual counselling should be part of the sexuality policy of the institution. Examples are: constant manipulation of the genitals, unprotected coitus, pregnancy, promiscuity, request to marry, overt sexual aggression, overt homosexual behaviour in inappropriate places, unsuccessful use of contraceptives, corporal punishment by parents for masturbation, exhibitionism or public masturbation, sexual abuse or use of another individual, sexual relations between an adult and a child.

There is a need to recognize that there are real problems concerning sexual counselling that do hinder progress, and require thought. The topics to be brought out into the open so they can be dealt with. Such discussion need not be discouraging nor provide ammunitition for those opposed to sexuality and the sexual expressions of mentally handicapped people. The goal in presenting these problems is strictly to help those doing sex counselling to foresee obstructions that might interfere with healthy outcomes.

How May One Become a Sex Counsellor?

Certainly not by only reading this book. The following information is given so that staff who find themselves in the position of counselling on sexual issues may be more effective.

The skills required are much the same for counselling anyone. However, the techniques differ. One must deal with the client's self-image, presenting levels of emotional, intellectual, and physical abilities as well as the capacity for communicating about sex. Each of these considerations may make the situation unique.

Annon's "PLISSIT Model" (1976) succinctly describes the type and intensity of requirements. He creates a pyramid of counselling services as follows:

1. *Permission*—The counsellor creates a non-threatening atmosphere where the client can talk about any aspect of sexuality. The counsellor must be comfortable with the topic, listen well and in a non-judgemental manner, and have a depth of knowledge regarding societal attitudes on the subject. (To some the use of the word permission may seem inappropriate, but its use as intended by Annon means "That's okay" "Nothing wrong with that," etc. . . . .)

2. *Limited Information*—Occasionally permission needs to be

augmented with information directly related to sexual concerns being presented. The task then becomes the eradication of myths, accomplished by the dissemination of information. This counsellor needs more relevant information than the "Permission" counsellor.

3. *Specific Suggestion*—This requires the counsellor to become more directive and assist the mentally handicapped person to set and reach concrete goals. Thus the counsellor should be an accomplished individual with experience, such as a family planning counsellor who gives concrete direction for using birth control methods.

4. *Intensive Therapy*—Only qualified counsellors are used to provide this service, "qualified" not only in sex counselling but also sex therapy. As mentioned before there are too few such counsellors.

It is possible that care-givers who understand the mentally handicapped can become sex counsellors on at least the first three of the PLISSIT Model levels. However, Kempton (1975b) spells out some additional skills. She recommends that such staff possess:

—sound basic knowledge of human sexuality and expertise in one or more aspects of sex counselling such as birth control, marriage, mental health, genetics, pregnancy, or sexual assault.

—an understanding of the common and special needs of the group of which the client is a member and an ability to relate to them. Clearly, the counsellor should know a good deal about the specific group to be counselled. A good counsellor of the mentally handicapped may be unprepared for the higher intelligence and verbal sophistication of many elderly and physically handicapped persons.

—the ability to discuss sexuality with ease and confidence.

—the ability to deal comfortably with the language of sex and to accept the clients' words until they can learn the technical terminology.

—an acceptance of sexuality as a positive force so that it will be unnecessary to struggle with unresolved personal conflicts, anxieties and tensions.

—an acceptance of varying sexual lifestyle and attitudes to avoid a negative subjectivity or a blocking of communications.

—a basic understanding of the legal and social issues involved in various aspects of the sexuality of special group members and the ability to counsel objectively on these issues.

—personality traits such as compassion, sense of humour, patience, perceptiveness, ingenuity and flexibility.

Conclusion

In providing counselling services we are taking one more step in the direction of normalization, the "utilization of means which are as culturally normative as possible in order to establish and/or maintain behavior and characteristics which are as culturally normative as possible" (Wolfensberger, 1972). This implies that mentally handicapped persons have the same rights and freedoms as anyone else living in a given society, including the enjoyment of sexual expression, sexual intercourse, marriage and procreation.

REFERENCES

Annon, J.S. (1976). The PLISSIT model: A proposed conceptional scheme for the behavioral treatment of sexual problems. *J.Sex.Educ.andTherapy 2,* 1, 1–15.

Bass, M.S. (1979). Contraception and Mentally Handicapped Persons. Paper presented at the Symposium on the Sterilization of Mentally Retarded Persons. National Institute on Mental Retardation of Canada, Toronto. May 14, 1979.

Caparulo, F. and Caparulo, B. (1979). Sexuality and the Handicapped: Whose Problem is it? *Sex Information and Education Council of United States Report 7,* 1 and 5.

Craft, A. and Craft, M. (1979). *Handicapped Married Couples.* London: Routledge and Kegan Paul.

Cruickshank, W. (1966). *Cerebral Palsy: Its Individual and Community Problems.* Syracuse, N Y: Syracuse University Press.

Goodman, L. (1973). Family Planning Programs for the Mentally Retarded in Institutions and Community. In: de la Cruz, F.F. and LaVeck, G.D. (eds). *Human Sexuality and the Mentally Retarded.* New York: Brunner/Mazel.

Goodman, L. (1975). The Sexual Rights for the Retarded—a Dilemma for Parents. In: Bass, M.S. and Gelof, M. (eds). *Sexual Rights and Responsibilities of the Mentally Retarded.* Proceedings of the conference of American Association on Mental Deficiency, Region IX, 1972 (revised edition).

Hall, J.E. (1974). Sexual Behavior. In: Wortis, J. (ed). *Mental Retardation (and Developmental Disabilities): An Annual Review.* Volume VI. New York: Brunner/Mazel.

Hall, J.E. (1975). Sexuality and the Mentally Retarded. In: Green, R. (ed). *Human Sexuality: A Health Practitioner's Text.* Baltimore: Williams and Wilkins.

Johnson, W. and Kempton, W. (1981). *Sex Education and Counseling for Special Groups.* Springfield, Ill.: Charles C. Thomas.

Kempton, W. (1975a). *Sex Education for persons with Disabilities that Hinder Learning: A Teacher's Guide.* Philadelphia: Planned Parenthood of Southeastern Pennsylvania.

Kempton, W. (1975b). Sex Education—a Co-Operative Effort of Parent and Teacher. *Exceptional Children 41,* 8, 531–35.

Mattinson, J. (1973). Marriage and Mental Handicap. In: de la Cruz, F.F. and LaVeck, G.D. (eds). *Human Sexuality and the Mentally Retarded.* New York: Brunner/Mazel.

Perske, R. (1972). The Dignity of Risk and the Mentally Retarded. *Mental Retardation 10*, 1, 25–7.

Wolfensberger, W. (1972). *The Principle of Normalization in Human Services.* Toronto, Canada: National Institute on Mental Retardation.

CHAPTER 5

The Parents' Viewpoint

Pauline Fairbrother

Let me first define the type of mentally handicapped people that I am writing about. It is those who are never allowed to venture out on their own, and therefore cannot live their own independent social and sexual lives. Should we attempt to educate these severely mentally handicapped young people and adults about sex? If the answer is 'yes', then having educated them to the best of our ability, and if they then put their education into practice, how do we counsel them? These are questions both parents and professionals have to face up to. But before we can do that, we have to resolve a fundamental issue. Do severely mentally handicapped people have any sexual needs or expectations? Many parents and professionals argue that they have not. "Why put ideas into their heads?" they say. What these well meaning people miss is that it is not into their heads that the ideas come, it is in their bodies, in their instincts. Apart from some aspects of growing up that I shall refer to later, it is not formal sex education that they need, but the help of people who are sensitive, open minded and observant of growing needs and of budding relationships who will give guidance and understanding.

"What they never have they will never miss" is another very sad little proverb that is all too often trotted out. It has been used to stop the path of progress for centuries. It was used to deny people decent housing, education and even butter. Unfortunately, unlike the need for butter or good homes or education, sexual needs are instinctive needs within all of us from the day we are born. To deny that they exist in any human is to court disaster and unhappiness. It seems logical once we accept the premise that all people have sexual needs to conclude that all people can cope better with those needs if they understand how they manifest themselves physically and emotionally. They need to know that they share these needs and feelings with everyone else. They need to know that they are not alone in their strange new emotions, their happiness and their misery. Everyone, and particularly mentally handicapped young people, needs to learn how to handle their emotions and what is acceptable and what is not.

Normal youngsters receive sex education. They might, if they are lucky, even receive sexual counselling on their problems. Then they are left to explore and experiment with relationships. Many mildly mentally handicapped youngsters will also follow this pattern. But the mentally handicapped people about whom I am concerned are not able to explore and experiment. If they do attempt to do so they can only do it with other people around, because they are never alone. And the other people, us, tell them that it is not socially acceptable. By the very nature of their handicap they are always overlooked, their lives are controlled and directed. So not only do mentally handicapped people need sex education and counselling but so too do we, the parents and the professionals, the 'overlookers'. Our attitudes must be examined and if necessary, undergo change if mentally handicapped people are ever going to have their sexual needs recognised and met. If we care enough then we have got to make it possible, for no one else will. Mentally handicapped people cannot make it possible on their own.

We tend to talk a great deal about the sexual problems of mentally handicapped people. But most of the problems that they have are imposed upon them by us. Why do parents in particular, become so depressed and worried at the first signs of sexual awareness, whether it is masturbation or giggling at someone of the opposite sex or becoming curious about their body? We should welcome joyously these signs as yet another manifestation of the *normality* of our son or daughter. The things that they have in common with the rest of us are far more numerous than the things that are different. An understanding of why parents feel this way should not only help them, but should also help professionals to understand them better.

The Relationship of Parent and Mentally Handicapped Child

To understand parents you have to understand their relationship with their mentally handicapped son or daughter. To understand their relationship you have to understand how that relationship grew and how it started. When a new baby is born the parents welcome it with joy and love and high expectations of its future. When the parents are told that their longed-for baby is not normal, is not as it should be, is handicapped, it is as if the baby they longed for and gave birth to has 'died'. They have to adjust to this new baby that is different. How well they adjust depends to a large extent on how they are told, what support they receive from their families, from professional people and from other parents of mentally handicapped children. What happens at that unreal, nightmarish time in their lives can colour their attitudes towards their child for the rest of his or her life. Those early days will be a big factor in their future acceptance or non-acceptance of their child becoming an adult with all that the word implies.

Other factors also mould parents' attitudes towards the sexual needs of their mentally handicapped son or daughter. For example there is the age of the parents and their generation's attitudes to sex; whether they can discuss it honestly and without embarrassment; whether their own experiences of sexual relationships have been happy and fulfilling, or unhappy and inhibiting. It also depends on whether there are other children in the family. Parents with normal children are more likely to make friends with couples of their own age who live a normal family life, often making these friends through their children. As their normal children grow up parents know, understand, and sometimes painfully, accept their adulthood and growing sexual needs. They are thus usually able to accept more naturally the adulthood and sexual needs of their mentally handicapped son or daughter. They have had experience of children growing up. If there is only one child, and that one is mentally handicapped, then parents become isolated and the only friends they make are those with mentally handicapped children also. It is usually the one-child parents who always refer to their son or daughter as their 'child'. I was recently at a Gateway Club and sitting next to a mother of an only son of 35. On being offered a piece of cake he forgot to say 'thank you'. His mother promptly reprimanded him, saying sharply, "If you do that again I shall smack you." To her, a loving, kind woman, he was and always would be a little boy.

The position in the family, if there are other children, can also be important. If the handicapped one is the youngest then the temptation to 'baby' him or her is very great. It happens in normal families, but then the youngest one will fight to be accepted as an adult, but the mentally handicapped person will not know how. The intelligence and occupation of parents can also colour attitudes. The intelligent, professional father usually has high expectations and ambitions for his child, particularly a son. Bitterness and resentment often leads to over protection. The only way he can accept that his son is never going to grow up in his image and expectation of him is to just not let him ever grow up at all. In contrast, parents who went to a special school themselves may not be unduly disappointed that their children go to the same school. Their expectations are not high and they happily accept their offspring as people, as children and later as adults. Most of us, of course, are somewhere in between those two extremes. But we all have some problems in coming to terms first with the handicap and then with the implications of sexuality.

However, all these factors are, I believe, of less importance than the way we were told that our child was mentally handicapped. It can influence our whole life. If we were told with sympathy and compassion, if we were informed about professional services available, if we were given guidance on how to manage, stimulate and help our child's development and if we were assured of support and relief, then we would have felt life was opening up again with a positive pattern, all was not lost. We would not feel, as so many of my generation felt, inadequate, isolated and hopeless. If we were also offered, right from the start, the understanding, support and hope from another parent of a mentally handicapped child, then we would probably have found ourselves well on the road to normality. In many parts of the UK some, or all, of the things that I have just listed are offered parents now, but sadly, the one of meeting another parent least often available. It is just not considered important. Doctors, health visitors and social workers declare that the parents are not yet ready to meet other parents. They make decisions for them, like we so often do for mentally handicapped people. Why don't these well meaning professional people try asking these new, bewildered parents if they would like the opportunity to discover that they are not alone? Of course, it is important that this is a service that should be built up on mutual trust between the local Society for Mentally Handicapped Children and Adults and the Hospital Authorities and local Social Services Departments. The parent volunteer must be acceptable by the hospital and local authorities.

It is my belief that apart from all the obvious benefits that this link-up of parents who share the same problems and heartbreak brings, there is a much quicker acceptance of the normality of their child. Everybody who has looked at the baby—the doctor, the nurses, the family and themselves—have all been very conscious of the handicap. But parents of mentally handicapped children or adults are used to mental handicap, they look for the baby, the person. It is always a joy to see a new baby arrive at an Opportunity Group or Mother and Baby Group. Mothers and helpers compete to hold it; everyone has a little cuddle and agrees that it is a beautiful baby, and everyone truly means it.

A mentally handicapped baby is not in isolation, it is part of a family. Its handicap affects all the family. They need to feel a united and ultimately, a normal family. They all need sympathetic help. By meeting other families, right from the beginning of the life of the mentally handicapped member of their family, the feeling of unreality is dispelled. If they are made to feel part of society and not rejected and if they are instructed on how to help their baby develop, then that child is not only less likely to be rejected but it will be loved in a normal, healthy way. If this happens then the attitude of the family and its friends towards the mentally handicapped member is more likely to be accepting of the right to adulthood.

The Adolescence Period

There are three emotionally charged times in the lives of parents of mentally handicapped children. One is when they are told of the handicap, and another is when they have to accept permanent residential care for their child or adult son or daughter, or when they face the question of what is to happen to their offspring when they, the parents, are dead. But what concerns us here is how parents come to terms with the adolescence of their handicapped child. We all, as parents, dream, even plan, for our children's future. We think of how proud we will be of their independence, standing on their own two feet and making a success of it. We look forward to our own independence, even if that is tinged with a little regret of the loss of the child that was. But we welcome the thought of holidays that suit us, being able to go out spontaneously and not having to get a sitter-in. We want to delight in their love for someone outside the family and in their marriage and we long for grandchildren. We all want immortality.

But if that son or daughter is mentally handicapped things are very different. We know that they are not likely to go into outside employment and if they do, the job is likely to be menial. We know that they are never going to be completely independent. We face the fact that our life is going to be different from 'the lives of our contemporaries. We are not going to enjoy the freedom of doing what we want, when we want. Everything must be planned. Sitters-in must still be found for our adult son or daughter, a much more difficult task when they are grown up. Mothers find it difficult to go out to work, for who is going to take their offspring to the doctor, the dentist, the hairdresser, the clothes shop and who is going to stay at home with them if they are ill? So not only is our life still full of responsibilites, but we suffer financially. All these things are painful and difficult things for parents to face at their son's or daughter's adolescence. Up till then their child has been a child, in both years and level of dependency, but this one will continue to need care and some protection, and so it is very easy to go on and on treating the growing person as a child. To many parents seeing them as a perpetual child is the only way that they can accept or cope with the handicap. It is the compensation. This attitude, though for different reasons, is not only confined to parents. It is often found in professionals working directly with mentally handicapped people. They see them as child-like and sexless. They, along with some parents, express the fear of "putting ideas into their heads".

Even amongst those parents and professionals who accept that mentally handicapped children become adults and have adult needs and desires, there is the very strong feeling that it is wrong to let these desires develop. There are the 'sterilizers' and the 'segregationists'. The 'sterilizers' want to see girls who show interest in boys sterilized. Mothers who are frightened of their daughters becoming pregnant see this as the only answer. I would perhaps have some sympathy for this argument if they say this as just a means of birth control and then make it possible for their daughters to lead a satisfying sexual life. But usually they do not, they hope that sterilization will quell all sexual desires. The 'segregationists' vary from the extremists, who want to keep males and females completely apart, to the more frequently encountered people who panic when they see a loving relationship developing between two mentally handicapped people. They assume that it must lead to either sexual intercourse or to frustration if the pair do not have the opportunity or perhaps the know-how to consummate their desires. Very often the 'segregationists'' views and beliefs are based on the false assumption, which is all too common in our modern world, that only sexual intercourse can satisfy sexual need. People talk of 'having sex' when they really mean having sexual intercourse. I think that this attitude is very unhelpful to mentally handicapped people, whose sexual needs often do not include sexual intercourse. I recently had a very worried mother ring me to ask if there was another ATC in the area. She wanted one for girls only because she was afraid of what might happen to her daughter if she was exposed to the desires of men! After assuring her that in the ten years that our ATC had been in existence I knew of no case of rape at the bench, I then went on to try to get her to actually put into words what she was worried about. When it was spoken about it all sounded rather silly, even to her. Basically she was frightened that her daughter would become pregnant because "everyone knew" mentally handicapped boys were not in control of themselves, and had strong desires for sexual intercourse.

Our Problem or Theirs?

The more that we examine our own attitudes, the more we must conclude that the sexual problems of mentally handicapped people are really our problems not theirs. We impose our problems, our attitudes, our beliefs, our prejudices, our fulfilment or lack of it onto mentally handicapped people. Because we have so much power over the destiny of these vulnerable persons, we intrude upon and shape their adult rights and needs. We direct and constantly observe their every move. We never allow them to be alone. We never allow them to explore relationships independently, to make mistakes and to find fulfilment. *They* do not need to change, all they need is loving guidance and the opportunity to fulfil themselves.

So if they do not need to change their attitudes towards their sexual needs, then we must. It has been interesting to note that whenever I have spoken to people, professionals or parents, about the sexual needs of mentally handicapped people, particularly if it is a residential course, my talk and the discussion afterwards, have always triggered off the need to talk about their own sexual problems, own experiences, own needs. I believe that many people need to go through this sometimes very painful exposure in order to start afresh looking at the subject in relation to mentally handicapped people. Given the right relaxed setting amongst those they know and trust, this discussion will happen spontaneously after the formal talk and questions. People seem to find it necessary to open up with their own personal happy or horror stories. They need to drop their guard, understand themselves, before they can talk honestly about helping others. The process may be very painful, but the sense of relief, or freedom, is well worth it.

Forums for Parental Discussion and Support

Venue and Participants

I think that this is the right place to look at the way that we discuss a sensitive subject such as sex. I am talking about the actual physical conditions under which we discuss them, not the content. Whatever the make-up of the group, whether it is just two people or ten (it really should not be more than ten, unless it is only the introduction to the subject), whether it is a group of professionals or a group of parents or a mixed group, or a group of mentally handicapped people, then the surroundings are of extreme importance. A comfortable room, with good, warm, not harsh lighting and comfortable chairs in a circle is important. It helps to have small coffee tables in front of the participants, not too high to create a barrier, but big enough to hide a little of themselves, so they do not start off feeling vulnerable. A glass of wine before the discussion helps to relax people. Whilst these groups should never be 'addressed' by someone, they should have one or two natural leaders prepared to start off the discussion. If it is a mixed professional and parent group then it is usually most effective if these two leaders each represent one of the two groups. Examples of problems or attitudes encountered from the public or at the ATC or in the family are often the best way to start it off, for in trying to solve a problem we find that we have to examine our attitudes.

How do we persuade these people to come together to discuss an embarrassing subject? Some professionals will come because they are genuinely concerned, and some will come because they feel that they should, it is their duty. It does not matter very much about the rest, they will usually follow the line of least resistance and accept the carrying out of new ideas. They will not help very much, but they probably will not hinder and they may eventually be convinced and enthusiastic. Mentally handicapped people are a captive audience and they are usually willing to participate in so far as they are able, and I am thinking here of the more articulate. The less articulate are going to have to rely on the full participation of parents and care staff. But here again it will only be a small percentage who will take part, but that percentage can be made higher by using a little guile. Do not ask them to come to discuss sexual problems. Ask them to come and have a glass of wine and a chat together about some of the anxieties that we all, parents and professionals, have about our mentally handicapped charges. Try meeting in a room over a pub or in a hotel, as long as it has the right sort of atmosphere that I described above. Do not meet in a private house; many people will feel at a disadvantage in someone else's home. Try not to meet at an ATC, unless everyone feels very much at home there, though a hostel may be the right place. But still only a few parents and a few professionals will participate. But they will be the ones who can change things. They will be the ones who can influence local councillors and ratepayers to provide living accommodation in the community and thus make close personal relationships possible. They will be in a position to give mentally handicapped people independence to explore relationships. They will be the ones who will talk to the public. They will be the ones who will pioneer ideas and thus bring about change. All the good changes and reforms have come about by the dedication and pressure of a small minority.

Ideally, parents and professionals should work together right from the time the diagnosis of mental handicap has been made. The Opportunity Group of mothers and babies in my borough talk about many things. They not only talk about the present, they look into and speculate about the future, sometimes about the future sexual development of their babies. I remember one such discussion in which a mother would not agree that her delightful little Down's Syndrome daughter would ever have sexual needs. Some few months later, when the little girl had started nursery school, I overheard another mother telling Patsy's mum about the performance every evening when her little boy got off the coach, how three year old Patsy and John had to be torn apart from their fond farewells. That was a loving, sexual, boy and girl relationship, a normal and natural event.

Choice of Discussion Leader

I suggested that a parent should be one of the people leading a discussion for three reasons. The first is that there is a strong bond between parents who have shared the same heartache, anxieties, joys and sorrows. Secondly, a parent can say things to other parents that a professional cannot. Parents know that another parent is talking from the experience of living with her mentally handicapped son or daughter. I use "her" quite deliberately, as I believe that it takes a remarkable father to speak on the subject of sexuality and be accepted without any feeling of discomfort by other parents. But most articulate mothers will be accepted by mothers, fathers and professionals without their motives being questioned. Thirdly, professionals because of their very professionalism, must view the subject soberly and solemnly. A parent can discard the solemnity surrounding the subject and can talk of it with love and warmth and humour. A sexual relationship, from touching and holding hands to sexual intercourse is a happy experience and this should be conveyed to mentally handicapped people. This does not mean that it should be viewed frivolously. It has to be thought about deeply, but not clinically.

Subjects for Discussion

We have looked at the setting and the discussion leaders. What do we discuss? Of course these groups are a forum for talking about many other areas of concern, such as the problems of siblings and how to prepare mentally handicapped people for their parents' eventual death and how to handle it when a parent actually dies (see Slater *et al* 1981). But these subjects, although of equal importance, are outside the scope of this book. Here, let us first consider subjects for the groups of parents and professionals, and later look at the groups of mentally handicapped people. We need to decide what we want to know. We are not seeking knowledge of something new, profound or clever. We are examining our own attitude to sex and our attitude (not what we say is our attitude, but what we really feel, which may not be the same) about the sexual needs and the sexual rights of mentally handicapped people. Are we frightened of our son or daughter, pupil, trainee or resident making a sexual relationship? What are we frightened of? What do we believe sex means to the mentally handicapped people whom we know? Are the needs of all mentally handicapped people the same? We should look at the mentally handicapped people the group know well. What signs of sexual awareness and needs have we noticed? The answers to this question can be particularly revealing if the group is composed of both parents and teaching or training staff. Very often our children will hide their feelings from us, but not from school or ATC staff. What sort of relationships do they form and do we allow them to develop freely? Do we ever leave them alone? How often do we tell them that it is not socially acceptable to indulge in petting at the Gateway Club, school, the ATC or the back of the coach? Do we then offer them an alternative, somewhere where it is socially acceptable? Do we and should we assume that like most normal young people, petting will lead to heavy petting and then to sexual intercourse? Maybe the needs of some mentally handicapped people are just to hold each other, to touch lovingly, to belong, to be special to someone outside the family, in other words, the basic human needs and rights of everyone to love and be loved? Maybe they want to sleep with each other because sharing the warmth of each other's bodies is a basic need? If the need is to make love and they do not know how, should we guide them? How will we know if they want guidance? Who will guide? Should they be encouraged to marry? What should be the criteria acceptable by us before we encourage marriage? Have they the right to bear children? What of the child's rights and future? Do the couple contemplating marriage understand the responsibility of bringing up a baby? For years my daughter, Di, used to tear at my heart strings saying that she wanted a baby until my youngest daughter had her first baby and came to visit us. Di then found that babies cry, babies wet themselves and other people's knees, that babies need a lot of patience and a lot of work. She has never expressed any desire to have a baby since. Should therefore all couples wanting babies be exposed to the hard facts of a couple of days with a young baby? What if they are not capable of independent living? Does that exclude them from marriage? Does that exclude them from a loving intimate relationship? What if, as a result of a loving, or just an experimental relationship, the girl is at risk of conceiving a child and we judge that it is not right for her or the future baby, to become pregnant? Who would be responsible for her use of contraceptives? Have we the right to decide on sterilization or abortion if she either objects or does not understand what is involved?

We need to look at the implications of physical development and prepare girls for menstruation. I remember believing that I had prepared Di by letting her see me and her eldest sister put on and take off sanitary towels, by telling her, very simply, what it was and that this happened to all girls when they grew up, and that it would happen to her. But all to no avail. She refused to tell anyone, or put on a sanitary towel herself when her period began. For about a year we had many problems. So how do we explain and prepare severely handicapped girls for menstruation? How do we cope with masturbation, particularly with boys. But let us remember it is not an exclusive form of comfort for boys only. It is no good telling a profoundly handicapped boy that, yes we know that it's nice and pleasant but, like going to the lavatory, it is only done in private. Many profoundly handicapped young men are taken to the lavatory by someone else, so that is not private. And, of course, if they live in an institution, privacy is usually the last thing they ever have. How do we prevent them doing it in the classroom, the workshop, or their living room, where not only is it embarrassing to watch, but it is also very unpleasant to have to clean up afterwards? How do parents cope with it? How do staff at schools and ATCs cope? How should they react to it? Are all these people left to manage as best they can or do they get any professional advice? Can we decide why they need to masturbate so often? Can the professionals, and here I mean the psychologist or psychiatrist, help us reduce the need?

With regard to subjects for discussion with mentally handicapped people themselves, my ATC has some very interesting recorded tapes. One of these tapes is about how they see themselves, their self-concept. It started spontaneously because some of them objected to riding in a mini bus labelled Merton Society for Mentally Handicapped Children. Firstly, they objected to the word 'children'. Secondly, they disapproved of 'mentally handicapped'. They recalled an incident in which one of the staff had been driving the bus and had annoyed the driver of another vehicle by his bad driving. The other driver, seeing the Society's name on the bus had implied that the name fully described the driver. The trainees asked the member of staff how he felt about being called mentally handicapped. Asked if they thought that they were mentally handicapped, they all said "No". They did realize that they had certain areas of difficulty and some limitations. They were all articulate people and could all travel on their own and therefore came into direct contact with unsympathetic members of the public. Because they were told by some members of the public that they were different, and even had their differences mocked, they were forced to look at themselves. My daughter, who is much more severely handicapped, is happy with the term 'mentally handicapped'. Her face lights up when she hears it. To her it means her friends and the things that Mum and Dad do. There is, I believe, a moral to be drawn from this. We must not conclude from what the more articulate mentally handicapped have said are their needs and their feelings, that these are necessarily the needs and feelings of all mentally handicapped people. But we must not conclude that the more severely handicapped have not got ambitions, needs and an image of themselves. It is much easier to persaude the more mildly handicapped to talk about themselves and each other, but the more severely handicapped need to express their feelings also. We need to find their areas of misunderstanding, why they behave in certain ways and what they feel about other people's behaviour, not only the behaviour of other mentally handicapped people, but ours as well. It will not be easy, but it may be very rewarding.

They need to be helped to discover who they are and what other people think of them and their behaviour. Trips outside the Centre or school where they meet the general public should be used for the basis of a discussion. Not just discussion on where they went, but on how people reacted to them and how they felt about some of the attitudes shown to them. They need to talk about what they would like to do and whether they really could do it. Of what they are frightened and what they get most joy from. They need to look at their relationships with other people, their family, staff and other mentally handicapped people. Words may not be enough, role play can be very useful to demonstrate how other people feel when they behave in certain ways or dress in a particular way or do not clean their teeth or bodies. They need to examine what love is to them and how they feel about someone they love or someone who loves them and how they should behave towards these people. They need an understanding and a pride in their bodies, even if those bodies are perhaps misshapen. They need to discuss and examine their bodies in private sessions with either a parent or a professional. Section drawings of parts of their bodies are no good, they do not mean anything to them. After all, how many people have ever seen a chopped off part of the body? Mirrors are essential in encouraging them to dress well, walk well, keep their faces and teeth clean, and to look pleasant.

This group should discuss masturbation. Why do they do it? Is it right to do it? Do they like seeing someone else in their group masturbating? They all know the word "sex", they hear it frequently and from many quarters. What is sex? What do they think that it is for? What is the connection between love and sex? What is marriage? Do they want to marry? What would they do if faced with the everyday, and the occasional big crises of marriage, and here play-acting is useful. Should a partner ever use physical violence on the other? How would they cope if one became ill? What would they do if someone they loved fell in love with someone else? Do they want children? Have they ever lived with a baby in the home? How are babies made? How would they cope with a sick or crying baby?

The areas of discussion are endless. But one thing is quite clear. Sex is not a subject to be discussed in isolation. It is part of life, it is the reason for the immortality of mankind. It is what we are, our self esteem, our manhood and womanhood.

Concluding Thoughts

If we accept that mentally handicapped people are people whose only deficiency is in their intellectual power, then we must accept their normal sexual needs. The more severely mentally handicapped are never alone, are not able to go out independently and find a home for themselves, or find a room or a garden or a street in which to walk and hold hands. They cannot do what every other normal youngster has the right and the opportunity to do. If we really mean what we say about helping them express their feelings then *we* must make it happen. They cannot make it happen themselves. If their relationships are going to blossom we have to do two things. Firstly we must provide the physical environment, homes in the community, group homes, homes with staff support, homes with minimum support and independent homes.

The next thing that we need to do is to persuade the general public, or at least those sections of the public that have power, members of parliament, local councillors, members of trade unions, political parties and women's organisations—that mentally handicapped people have needs and rights. We cannot provide houses in the community if they are sited amongst disapproving ignorant people. I mean ignorant in the nicest possible way. Ignorant people are ignorant because they do not know. Once they know they are no longer ignorant. It is up to us to dispel that ignorance.

If mentally handicapped people are to live fulfilled lives, we, parents and professionals, have to make it happen.

REFERENCES

Slater, J. Fitzpatrick, S. and Carrins, D. (1981). Helping to Overcome Fears for the Future. *Social Work Today, 12,* 30, 11–12.

CHAPTER 6

Health, Sex and Hygiene Education in Special Schools

June McNaughton

The World Health Organisation's survey of 16 European countries shows that in Czechoslovakia, East Germany, Sweden and Denmark, sex education is compulsory but in Greece, Turkey and Algeria, it is rare—though not actually prohibited (Isaev, 1979). In the United Kingdom sex education is officially approved but not sanctioned by legislation and is at the discretion of the head teacher in every school. The report further stated that the sex education curriculum is limited almost everywhere to anatomy, menstruation and prevention of V.D.

It is not only in Europe that curriculum development in this area has been delayed. Paul Gebhard (1980), one of the foremost American researchers into sexual behaviour, states that

> Society has in the main grudgingly accepted the need for some sexual instruction prior to marriage. . . . There was and still is great resistance to sex education below the college level. Many otherwise reasonable people cling to the idea that children are sexless innocents who would never have a sexual thought or impulse unless some adult has spoiled their purity with premature knowledge.

And yet the sex of an individual is an integral part of personality. One of the first questions asked after a child's birth is 'is it a boy or a girl?' The birth of a son evokes quite different feelings from the birth of a daughter. Gender affects the mode of dress, behaviour, interests and the expectations and demands of parents and society.

When realising how slow society has been to consider sexuality as an important part of human personality and behaviour, it is not surprising that the rights of retarded individuals to attain knowledge of their sexuality has been neglected.

Special schools considering the development of programmes of sex education face two problems. First, the wide range of individual variations amongst the educationally subnormal in special schools

110

which makes it difficult to make statements which apply universally to all pupils. The ESN(M) (EMR) living at home have different needs from the SSN (TMR) or those living in residential schools. The former may well marry and have children while the latter are not encouraged in this direction. Even amongst the ESN(M) pupils the variance in ability, development and living situations precludes a single set of objectives. Some may be physically immature; others whilst retarded mentally may be physically well-developed. Cultural differences may add a further dimension.

The second problem is that sex education has no traditional educational model about which there is a consensus of opinion. As a society we have not given sex education in schools a high priority. One argument used to explain this has been that it is 'the responsibility of parents'. However, Christine Farrell in *My Mother Said . . .* (an assessment of young people's sexual knowledge, attitudes and behaviour based on interviews with 1500 sixteen- to nineteen-year-olds) pointed out that while the majority of parents feel they ought to play the main part in imparting knowledge in this area, only a minority actually do (Farrell, 1978). Meanwhile, schools hesitate and children pick up information or misinformation elsewhere.

Teachers in special schools have different expectations about their pupils' sexuality and potential maturity from teachers in mainstream schools. Everyone expects children of normal intelligence to grow into mature, independent and responsible adults; indeed the development of autonomy and maturity is the acknowledged aim of British schools. The mentally handicapped are, however, by definition, expected to have a lower potential for future independence. How then should and can they be prepared for adulthood—indeed what does adulthood mean in this context?

As with any aspect of education concerned with social behaviour, the aim is to equip pupils to become socially responsible members of their community with an understanding and acceptance of their own identity and the ability to form successful relationships. Sex education is best integrated into the wider setting of Health Education rather than isolated instruction but health education itself has also suffered from the lack of a traditional model or clear definition. By some it is still perceived as sex and hygiene teaching, an attitude lightheartedly summed up as 'dirty feet, dirty heads and the dirty bits in between'.

A broader definition of health education has been provided by the Schools Council, an independent body which carries out research on curricula and teaching methods. The Schools Council Project: Health Education 5–13 produced two teachers' guides embodying their rationale (1977 (a) and (b)). The Project's interpretation of the word 'health' was very wide, embracing physical health and hygiene, emotional and social development. Four important points formed the cornerstone of this rationale:

(1) A conviction that health education is largely concerned with the behaviour of individuals and groups.
(2) That behaviour is, in part, developmental and as such is rooted in the process of primary and secondary socialisation.
(3) That to be effective health education must form a positive part of socialisation and, therefore, be seen as an integral part of formal as well as informal education.
(4) That health education must be organised and continuous.

In other words, Health Education is neither to be seen as a once and for all experience, nor should it be left to crop up in a haphazard way, but should be seen as an integral part of the school curriculum.

Health and sex education, like all education, occurs at three levels: incidental, experiential and formal. In referring to health education in schools, we mean *planned* experiences but the process of socialisation has given all children an incidental education before they begin school. From birth a child builds up ideas about himself and others, about human warmth and love, about the roles of men and women. The retarded child is exposed to many of the same experiences as other children and his physical growth follows the same pattern—though the timing may vary. However, the ESN child may not have the same opportunities to develop, and discover, until it is socially unacceptable. For instance the early adolescent stage of peer group interaction and 'giggle' contact with girls may for many ESN boys be prevented until a stage of development when such behaviour may cause some concern.

In order to see health and sex education as a developing process, we need to think of health behaviour in terms of a 'career'. Often we concentrate our efforts and resources at the point at which the sex 'crisis' appears. We see the child growing physically into an adult and respond to the crisis by asking 'when should we begin sex education?' However, before this there has been an accumulation of influences from family, peers and the media. Consequently health education needs to reflect this and begin early. Of course the nature of the teaching will be of a different order at different times, reflecting the developmental stage of the pupils. What we need to think of is a curriculum which 'spirals' to coincide with the growth and progress of children (see Fig. 1).

Developing a School Programme

There are no short cuts to programme planning in health and sex education. Before launching a school programme it is essential for the success of the venture that certain considerations are taken into account. It is important for instance that with a subject as sensitive as sex education that teachers feel secure in what they are doing. Sex education touches on some fairly controversial areas. If teachers are to feel comfortable, time is required to explore the issues involved and consider their relevance to the everyday work of the school. There are also organisational implications. The school should, therefore, organise a planning group to consider the task.

In small special schools this will involve teachers and care staff. The person leading this first stage process has a crucial part to play and should, therefore, be a senior member of staff—probably the Head or Deputy. Since this is a curriculum development exercise the leader needs an understanding of the philosophy involved, an idea of its relevance to the work of the school and status within the school to implement new curriculum development.

After the establishing of a curriculum development group a four-stage process is involved:

CLARIFICATION—PLANNING—IMPLEMENTATION—EVALUATION

The possible questions which need to be answered within these four processes are dealt with below:

A. CLARIFICATION—the Establishment of Curriculum Objectives

(1) What are the nature and aims of health education?
(2) What is its place in the curriculum?
(3) What content?
(4) What is the role of parents?

A1. *The Nature and Aims of Health Education*
No-one can take away from schools the task of deciding what to

113

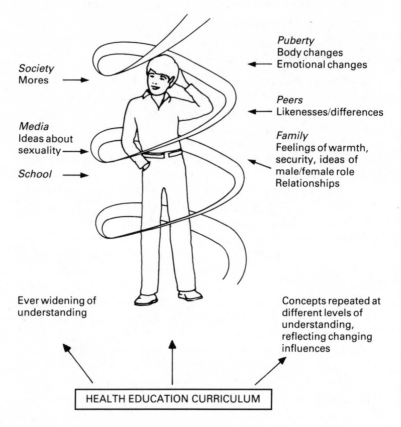

Figure 1: The framework and fundamental concepts of Health Education.

teach and how. Health Education must be tailored to the philosophy of each individual school and the needs of its pupils. For all schools the most important thing to cultivate is a sense of personal identity and self respect with possible concentration on two main strands, 'Knowing about Myself' and 'Knowing about Others'. Through health education we hope to make pupils more able and competent to manage themselves and their lives. Successful management demands self confidence, a positive self image and the ability to relate to others.

The development of a positive self concept relies not on the use of a particular unit of work but is influenced by the experience of the pupil in and out of the school—in particular the ethos of the school and the teaching methods in Special Schools. The nature of pupils' limitations may be the cause of experiences which contribute to a negative view of Self. Meeting with tasks beyond his capability, lack of opportunity to assert himself, all contribute to the picture the handicapped pupil has of himself. Special schools meet this challenge intuitively every day but a fresh look at their approaches can help to keep this a conscious effort.

It is sometimes argued that slow learning children are in many ways 'different' and that there should, therefore, be differences in the programmes provided for such pupils. However, if there are to be differences between the way we approach health education for the mentally handicapped and for other pupils, we need to be clear about the reasons for such differences. Certainly there should be no difference in philosophy. If we are to accept mentally handicapped pupils as growing and developing people like any other pupils, we cannot set absolute limits for them—although in individual cases a realistic appreciation of their total situation sets some parameters for their development. It is impossible, however, to accept any suggestion of different sets of ethics for those with handicaps. At this level the aims of health education apply to all.

> The same hopes of developing an individual able to operate as efficiently as possible within this environment, to contribute as well as he can to the community and to show appropriate concern and consideration in his relationships with others, might be held for all children. The extent to which these or other aims might be realised is determined by the responsiveness of the child to learning experiences and the skill with which they are devised. (D.E.S., 1975).

The aims point the general direction but at a subsequent level of

115

determining the outcomes and short-term objectives full account needs to be taken of the pupils' abilities and handicaps. Having set the horizons, continual smaller decisions have to be made about the routes to these objectives.

A2. *Determining the place of health education in the curriculum*
The place of the health and sex programme is within the personal and social education of the school. Some schools already have 'Life Skills', 'Social Competence' or other such programmes of personal development and these offer a proper context for health teaching. These courses may operate throughout the school, or be specifically geared to leavers' groups. If the programme is focussed on one age group only, ways to extend the work to other pupils can be sought.

A3 *Curriculum Content: What should we teach?*
While for the severely handicapped a careful selection of priorities amongst content areas is necessary, for moderately handicapped students the content areas to be covered should not differ greatly from those planned for mainstream pupils, although starting points will vary.

As well as the obvious differences in cognitive ability, mentally handicapped pupils also have much *in common* with other pupils. Though a pupil's mental age may be comparable to that of a child half his age, in no way can we equate his social experiences, his physical development or his rights and responsibility with those of the younger child. Much of what he is required to learn and come to terms with is the same as for any other pupil of similar age—but the way he learns is very different.

At each age there are 'developmental tasks' which *all* children have to come to terms with as they grow, regardless of academic ability, therefore content areas for slow learners may not be significantly different. It is the depth of study and the methods which will vary. Also the outcomes of the programme will need consideration. The desired outcomes for those who are likely to live independent lives in the community will be different from those who cannot be expected to achieve independence. For example, education about intercourse and childbirth have a different context for those unlikely to marry

Advice for Special Schools on health education is sadly lacking. *Health Education in Schools* published by the Department of Education and Science (1973) has only one passing reference to

116

Special Schools and no guidelines exist. In the absence of an educational model for special schools, an examination of programmes for mainstream health education may offer some suitable guidelines. The content of the SCHEP 5-13 guides, for instance, reflects the physical and emotional growth of pupils and thus indicates the educational needs at their successive developmental stages (see Figures 2 and 3).

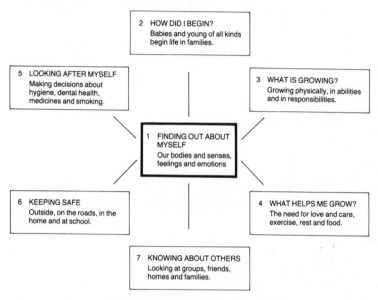

Figure 2: *All About Me* (5–8 years)

The Schools Council has now funded a three-year extension to this mainstream project so that the materials can be adapted for use with slow learning pupils. The Extension Project, due to be completed in December 1981, is adopting the same rationale and content areas as the 'parent' project, but the approaches and methods will take full account of the pupils' learning levels.

EARLY YEARS. For all children the starting point is the establishing of a self identity. This, and the control of the body and its basic functions, provides a springboard for later work.

Establishing a Self Concept involves considering self awareness to provide the basis for the self concept theme which is threaded at different levels through the rest of the work.

Looking at babies offers a starting point for introducing early work on sex education putting it into its natural context and stressing the

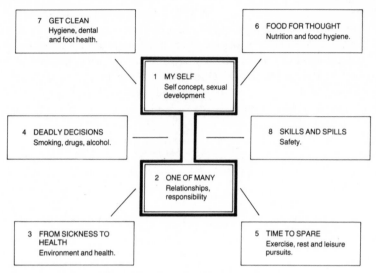

Figure 3: *Think Well* (9–13 years)

need for teachers to be aware of how much information children already have. Most children begin school with an idea of their sexual identity (boy/girl). They need to learn a basic body vocabulary and gradually acquire simple concepts such as:

– Living things come from living things.
– Like comes from like.
– Babies need care, love and protection.
– Human babies grow inside their mother before they are born.

Growth. During the early years it is valuable if children can grasp the concept of themselves as growing, developing individuals. This is not an easy idea to grasp, but will add meaning to work on food, rest, exercise and safety.

Relationships. A feeling and understanding for relationships with others also relies on self-awareness and self-confidence. The important ideas to establish are sharing, helping and belonging.

MIDDLE YEARS. As pupils approach puberty the physical changes that gradually take place in their bodies need to be explained and discussed. Some instruction should coincide with these changes, though girls in particular will need preparation in advance. Changes can cause alarm in the uninformed. The retarded need considerable help in coping with the changes in feelings and the changes in

118

relationships which occur with this growing up. The transition to adulthood can be a stormy period for the average teenager but for the handicapped there may be further complications when a child matures physically either earlier or later. Children need to try to come to terms with the differences and similarities between them. For example:

- Physical differences.
- Similarities and differences in feelings.
- Families
- Likes and dislikes, e.g. class preferences of food, activities, etc.
- Feelings about what makes other people happy, unhappy, sad, etc.
- Friendships.

Health teaching in other areas can reflect the pupils' growing responsibility for their own self-care and take into account the increasing number of situations involving choices and decisions.

UPPER SCHOOL. Many ESN schools already organise leavers' courses which include child-care and parentcraft courses. These courses are excellent in preparing pupils for their adult role. However, we must guard against placing personal relationships only in the context of childbirth and child-care. Pupils need help in forming relationships before marriage and in learning acceptable 'dating' behaviour, and should not be left with the idea that marriage and childbirth are the only measures of success in the adult world. This limits the choices which they see open to them as they grow up.

At this stage emotions can be very powerful and children need help in coming to terms with them. Pupils are usually very much aware of pressures to conform often to the peer group. Education should be directed to helping children to cope with these pressures. Retarded children can be very compliant and this has implications for all kinds of behaviour. For instance, it makes them vulnerable in situations where there is a possibility of exploitation of any kind.

A4. *What about Parents?*

Parental attitudes of health and sex education vary but most parents welcome help. Watson (1980) found that parents of ESN(M) children tended to think their children were lacking in sex knowledge and a high proportion wanted their children to receive sex education at school or both school and home.

Most parents are happy for the school to take the initiative in sex education. As mentally handicapped children approach adolescence many parents become anxious about what lies ahead and some admit that it is hard for them to talk about sex to their children.

A parents' meeting at a special school can be a good forum for their worries to be aired. The school may make this an occasion to show films or slides which form part of the teaching programmes and discuss how these are to be used. Some schools seek parental permission to give sex education, whereas others feel that while good relations and co-operation are important there is no need for such a formal approach. Many feel that sex education, though an important part of the school social curriculum is, nevertheless, a part not essentially different from any other, and to single it out and isolate it by asking permission is to take it out of its proper context in the curriculum.

Whatever approach is adopted by the school, the need for sympathetic understanding between school and home remains. Understanding and support from parents brings many benefits including that of protecting teachers from ill-informed and unwarranted criticism. Where objections do occur it is useful to point out that schools are not the only educators. No child can be shielded from the influences of peers, the media and other environmental factors; we cannot stop their receiving sex education *of a kind*.

Reaching parents is, in some instances, difficult. The wide catchment area of special schools, or the memories—not always positive—of their own schooldays may keep many parents away from the school, but the benefits to school and home make the effort worthwhile.

B. PLANNING

(1) What is the existing provision?
(2) What are the priorities?
(3) What are the starting points?
(4) How do we deal with problems?

B1. *What is the existing provision?*

While perceptions of health education might differ, all schools are usually engaged in some kind of health/sex education though they do not always see it as such. One way to explore this is to provide teachers with a grid using a simple checklist and ask them to check the topics they cover in the course of their work. The information can then be collated and put onto a master grid.

Sophisticated grids can be drawn up using the lists such as Figures 4 and 5 but a simple example illustrates the intention of the exercise:

	Under-standing ourselves	Myself and others	Protecting our health	Lifestyle and health	Food enjoyment and health	Safety
Class 1	My body The senses	Things I like	Self care	Our day	What do we eat? Feeding	Don't touch!
Class 2	How did I begin? etc. Mothers and babies	Homes and families	Exercise	Things we like to do	Trying new foods etc.	Road Safety
Class 3	Feelings & emotions etc.	My friends	Keeping clean	Using our time etc.	Eating habits	Play safely
Class 4	How we grow	Learning about others	Our medicines	Exercise etc.	Food we like	Accidents

Such information plotted onto a master grid can provide useful data concerning the school and what is being attempted and can also be used for spotting gaps in the existing provision. This may provide a starting point for the development of health teaching.

What the grids will not illustrate is to what extent the contributions to the health education curriculum rely on chance situations arising during the everyday life of the school, as opposed to the deliberately planned formal inputs. Further, the incidental or 'hidden' curriculum which pupils experience through the ethos of the school will not be revealed. However much is planned in the way of formal lessons in health education this incidental education will still crop up. Some teachers believe that all health and sex education should be given incidentally 'as the need arises' or 'spontaneously' or 'in answer to questions'. This approach may, however, prove inadequate on several grounds. The retarded ask few questions and exhibit little curiosity. Unlike the 'normal' pupils who create 'teachable moments' by their questions, the slow learners require the skilful setting up of the learning situation with planned, structured lessons in addition to the informal approach. Where

Figure 4

EXAMPLE OF A CURRICULUM GRID

Curriculum survey 5–8 year olds   *Form A*

Class teacher's name

Year/age group

In the list below you will find a large selection of topics.

So that we can see if this forms a useful developmental pattern in our school, please will you tick those you have (or hope to) cover during the current school year. (Cover = taught to the majority of children.)

Finding out about myself	*Tick here*
The senses	
What do I look like?	
About my body	
Emotions	
How did I begin?	
Baby animals	
Human babies	
How babies are cared for	
Growth	
How our shape and size changes	
How we develop	
How our responsibilities grow	
What do we need for growth?	
Love and care	
Exercise	
Rest	
Food	
Looking after myself	
Hygiene	
Care of teeth	
Illness	
Smoking	
Safety	
Road safety	
Other aspects of outdoor safety	
Home and school safety	
Knowing about others	
How we get on together in school	
My friends	
Homes and families	

Reprinted from *Professional Development Workshop Manual* (1979)
The Health Education Council/TACADE.

EXAMPLE OF A CURRICULUM GRID   Figure 5

Curriculum survey 9–16 year olds   *Form B*

In the list below you will find a selection of health education topics.

So that we can see if this forms a useful developmental pattern in our school, please will you tick those covered in the relevant age groups, during the *current* school year. Include those already taught and those which will be taught in the remainder of the year. (Cover = taught to the majority of children.)

	Year (Please fill in)			
Understanding ourselves Awareness of self How we relate to others Feelings and emotions Growth and development Sex education				
Myself and others How others expect us to act How we make decisions The family Friendships Heterosexual relationships Other relationships Who moulds us—groups —media				
From Sickness to Health What is illness? Spread of disease Cure of disease				
Things we take Smoking Drinking and alcohol Other drugs and medicines				
Time Using time Exercise Rest Leisure				
Food Eating habits Keeping food clean Choice of food Vitamins Advertising and food Food and the body—growth/repair				
Cleanliness General hygiene Teeth Clothes, shoes, feet				
Safety Road safety Home safety Leisure safety Finding out about accidents Swimming Emergency aid First aid				

Reprinted from *Professional Development Workshop Manual* (1979)
The Health Educational Council/TACADE.

instances do crop up unexpectedly, without premeditation the teacher is left to deal with important topics 'off the cuff' instead of in a carefully prepared situation. This is difficult enough in normal schools but extremely difficult when teaching slow learners.

B2. *What are the Priorities?*

A curriculum survey of the nature mentioned above will reveal what *is* going on in the school. This needs to be matched against the question of what *ought* to be going on. One way to gauge the priorities amongst the staff is to ask teachers to use the same lists to rate each topic for its degree of importance. Outside opinion could also be sought. In doing this teachers should bear in mind the "Spiral Curriculum". Pupils may appear too young or too handicapped for some topics but there is a need to anticipate future needs rather than chase problems.

An examination of the school 'grid' can reveal whether the most highly rated topics are being given most weight. Examination might also show gaps in provisions which point to planning priorities or reveal topics which are not being introduced at an early stage of development.

B3. *Starting Points*

Before allocating extensive resources to the programme, a pilot programme for a limited term can test out the curriculum. This will allow teachers to gain a measure of expertise and allow the school to see if their planning is on target.

An alternative starting point could be a review of resources and the piloting of a selection of these.

B4. *Problems*

However much agreement there is among staff about the broad principles, there are bound to be topics which create uncertainty or disagreement. Some areas such as masturbation, homosexuality, V.D., incest and abortion, are so sensitive that their place in a school educational programme is a matter on which opinions differ. Society as a whole has yet to make up its mind where it stands on some issues and yet expects schools to cope with the controversies.

Again, as with other aspects of the curriculum, it is the needs of the pupils which decides the issues. Information on matters such as sexually transmitted disease should be given for protective purposes. Instruction need not be detailed, but focus on the symptoms, how it is contracted and the need to seek medical advice.

Homosexuality is a topic which can cause concern. Popular terms for homosexuals are frequently bandied about in quarrels as insults by some retarded pupils—often with little understanding of the meaning of the words. The subject is frequently the focus of silly jokes—which media stereotypes have, sadly, done much to popularise. The behaviour of some of the retarded appears to indicate a preference for friendships with the same sex; it is advisable not to read too much into this behaviour. All children go through the stage of 'crushes' on people of the same sex. When this stage is delayed it can give cause for comments which would not have arisen at an earlier age. Also the retarded lack many of the opportunities for making friends which normal pupils have.

Schools may be in a quandary as to how to approach this topic. Though films or slides may be available, discussion about friendships in general and ample opportunities of mixing with a wide range of young people is the best focus of the instruction. Through talk about friendships the teacher can guide the discussion to take account of the requirements of the pupils and turn the focus towards particular problems.

If sexuality is denied all natural expressions of sexual behaviour are construed as problems. This is particularly the case with masturbation. However, it is not masturbation itself which is a problem, but only when it is inappropriate, e.g. done at the wrong time or place. Ideas that such behaviour is 'dangerous' or harmful should be dispelled, but pupils can be helped to be responsible about other people's feelings and learn that some behaviours are personal and private.

C. IMPLEMENTATION
    (1) Who teaches?
    (2) What methods?
    (3) Do we have the resourses?

C1. *Who teaches?*
The incidental nature of health/sex education means all staff are involved in some way, but some teachers may feel uncomfortable about being involved in the more formal teaching of the more sensitive areas. Generally it is thought that no pressure should be brought on them. The availability of well designed materials is

crucial here. Some teachers who cannot visualise themselves being involved in teaching new or sensitive topics can often realise the relevance of health and sex education to their work if the approach and starting points are right.

Many teachers feel that lessons about sex education should be organised on an individual basis. Certainly provision for individual counselling is desirable but class and group discussion is a useful teaching approach for many topics. Except for a few areas such as menstruation, which is often easier to discuss with an all-girls group, the groups can be mixed. In the case of menstruation girls need particular help with self-care and hygiene problems connected with periods and this is more appropriately done in a small counselling group. Boys, too, may benefit from an opportunity for counselling in a small group. Boys' worries at puberty may include wet dreams and a counselling group can give the teacher an opportunity to reassure them about the normality of these occurrences and the chance to avoid confusion between wet dreams and bed-wetting.

C2. *What methods?*

Having proceeded by stages to planning the curriculum two further questions which need to be answered are: 'What methods? What materials and resources are available?'

We need some degree of consistency between the educational theory underpinning the teaching of health education and the methods employed with slow-learners.

If health education is to be viewed as a process then teaching must take into account not only the acquisition of facts, but also feelings and skills. If we accept that the task is to work towards a health autonomy in pupils—within the constraints of their physical, emotional and intellectual development—then we need also to help them make decisions about their lives and health. It is not just a matter of teaching pupils how to put on clothes, but of helping them to choose what to wear, not simply of training pupils to feed themselves in an acceptable manner, but of helping them to make choices about what to eat. In our anxiety to protect the handicapped we often end up telling them what to do and how to behave.

Because of their limitations we must accept the responsibility of deciding for them for much longer than for normal children. Of course protection is needed but the whole thrust of the work should be towards giving personal meaning to the topics so that children can think in terms of their *choices* rather than the decisions of the teacher. To this end, facts need to be presented in their social context. For example, the biological facts of intercourse and reproduction need to be given a social context which has meaning and relevance to the pupils concerned. Without a context with which they can identify sex education will have no meaning and little value.

All pupils bring with them to the health education lesson a background of previously acquired attitudes and facts—some of them inaccurate. One way to ensure that the lesson has meaning is to begin by eliciting what the pupils already know and feel about the topic. Ideas, including misinformation, can then be explored without loss of face. ESN pupils are often very glib in using vernacular terminologies, but discussion may reveal that they are unclear about the real meanings of such vocabulary.

The materials for eliciting information need to be clear and unambiguous and the language of instruction should take into account the pupils' own vocabulary. Some teachers may feel inhibited in using the students' vernacular language, but the important thing is for the teacher to ensure that the children know what is being talked about. Ways must be found to link the children's own words to the more socially acceptable words.

It is not easy to prepare slow learners to enable them to make decisions in social situations. Many of the opportunities which normal teenagers have of learning to mix with others is denied them. In many cases the mentally handicapped are poorly equipped for the social freedom they may later experience in the community. Because of their greater vulnerability they are afforded more protection which limits the opportunities still further.

In view of this many schools feel that encouraging moral behaviour must rate high in their aims. Teachers will, of course, wish to emphasise the place of loving relationships as part of marriage and other stable relationships. Teachers also need to be aware that their own experiences and attitudes may be different from those of their pupils. Those able to live independent lives after school will take their place in a society that is ambivalent in its attitudes relating to sexuality and the young school leaver may be particularly vulnerable to sexual advances so that moral guidance alone will be no protection. Slow learners need sensitive guidance about the consequences of their behaviour and their responsibilities. Role play or socio-drama offer a useful medium to explore and prepare for future situations.

Morals are culture-specific, but the important issues in our society are all capable of being grasped by ESN(M) pupils:

– no one must use a child sexually
– no one must commit a sexual act with another adult if the adult is unwilling
– no one need allow another person to use them sexually
– all sexual behaviour involving the genitals should be done in private
– physically mature people risk starting a baby if they have sexual intercourse and do not use contraception. No one should conceive children they cannot look after and provide for.

C3. *Do we have the resources?*

There is a dearth of good health education material which has been designed specifically for the mentally handicapped. Because of this teachers may need to make imaginative use of material which was not designed primarily for health education. Language development kits can be a useful source of material. These kits often have material which can lend itself to work relating to body parts, to emotions, to work about food and eating and particularly to work about relationships and families. Films and slides produced for mainstream pupils can sometimes be used if the sound-track is replaced by the teachers' own commentary.

Frequently teachers will be thrown back on their own resources. Often these can be simple and effective—clarity is the basic criteria. For instance, a set of pictures cut from magazines can be used to stimulate discussion about family relationships. Teaching about a variety of topics could emerge from this by the teacher asking questions about the likely roles, behaviour, etc., of the people. Topics such as pregnancy, getting married, could develop from this discussion. Teenage dolls can be similarly used.

D. EVALUATION

(1) Measures of success

D1. *Measures of success*

"You can't teach them anything. They will still go out and get pregnant." This comment, made by a teacher from an ESN(M) school and quoted by Watson (1980) sums up the doubts of many teachers. What measures of success can we look for? Many teachers feel that since the school is but one of the many influences its effect must be limited. "At this ESN(M) school it is our experience that sex education has a limited value. The majority of our pupils will behave in accordance with the mores of their social group" (Watson 1980). Certainly schools frequently face demands to solve problems they did not create or cope with influences over which they have no control. The pupils living in the community cannot be insulated from its effects. But it is too easy to dwell on the rather negative aspects. There are more positive reasons for considering health and sex education besides the preventive reasons such as avoiding unwanted pregnancies or V.D. The pupils' sexuality is an integral part of personality and an essential element in the adult role. In preparing pupils for the future teachers must not discount or ignore this sexuality.

What of the Future?

What future are we preparing for? There is no one answer. Most of the moderately handicapped will take their place in society; many will marry and have children just like other people. This may be one of the few areas where they achieve success. For the severely handicapped this is less easy to predict, but we must ensure that the education we provide is an enabling one not a limiting one, and try to give the pupils the ability to cope with new situations. An education which helps a pupil to understand himself and his feelings and makes him sensitive to the feelings and needs of others is of more value than one which teaches a boy to read but not how to interpret the reactions of other people or teaches a girl to handle money without knowing her own value.

This is the challenge of curriculum development which can lead to a re-evaluation of what special schools and their teachers are trying to do.

REFERENCES

Department of Education and Science (1973). *Handbook of Health Education,* third impression, London: HMSO.
Department of Education and Science (1975). *Educating Mentally Handicapped Children.* Pamphlet 60. London: HMSO.

Farrell, C. (1978). *My Mother Said . . .* London: Routledge & Kegan Paul.

Gebhard, P.H. (1980). Sexuality in the Post-Kinsey Era. In: Armytage, W.H.G., Chester, R. and Peel, J. (eds.). *Changing Patterns of Sexual Behaviour.* London: Academic Press.

Health Education Council/TACADE (1979). *Professional Development Workshop Manual.*

Isaev, D.N. (1979). Learning About Sex. *World Health*, October, pp 20–23.

Schools Council (1977a). Health Education 5–13: *All About Me.* Sunbury-on-Thames: Nelson.

Schools Council (1977b). Health Education 5–13. *Think Well.* Sunbury-on-Thames: Nelson.

Watson, G. (1980). Sex Education Surveyed. *Special Education: Forward Trends,* 7, 3, 11–14.

See also: McNaughton, J. for the Schools Council (1983) *Fit for Life.* London: Macmillan Educational Ltd.

CHAPTER 7

Why is it such a Big Secret?
Sex Education for Handicapped Young Adults

Hilary Brown

Many handicapped young people face the emotional and physical
changes of adolescence amidst a conspiracy of silence from those of
us 'in the know'. Their limited ability to understand is thus compounded and their status as young men and women in our society
left in question. They enter our Further Education Colleges and
Adult Training Centres ill-equipped to make sense of their feelings
and behaviour, or to respond to those in whose company they pass
their time.

In this chapter I shall be drawing on my experience in groups at
the Spastics Society's Dene College, a two-year residential programme for young people who are both physically and mentally
handicapped. I shall discuss the level of personal and sexual awareness in such a group and the problems this raises for them, and
others like them. I shall look at ways of sharing simple information
about human sexuality, and describe the effect such information has
on these hitherto sheltered young people. We shall also consider
current moves in Adult Training Centres to include sex education as
a facet of social skills training and practical steps which can be taken
to set up a programme in this context.

Information about human sexuality and sexual behaviour is a
vital part of any programme which seeks to prepare mentally
handicapped people for life in the community. The issues and
anxieties which they raise testify to the need for honesty and support
from those of us who purport to care. Moreover when we include
them as equals in the 'big secret' we convey adult status and worth,
thus enabling them to value themselves and to see each other as a
source of joy and understanding. As such I view sex education as a
very positive experience and not one to be feared.

The level of awareness

A survey of students entering the Spastics Society's two further education colleges in 1979 showed this group of multiply-handi-capped young people to be largely isolated from sexual information (Brown, 1980). Only one-quarter, the more able of the group, had received any kind of sex education in school and without exception, they were unwilling or unable to talk to their parents about their feelings or experiences—indeed many did not think their parents knew about sex. Moreover, critically, only one young man in our survey of 50, mentioned having talked about sex in a group of his peers.

A simple questionnaire was administered to test the accuracy of information which had filtered through. It was limited to the more publicly acceptable images. Most students knew that babies grow inside their mothers and are fed at the breast, but few knew what men have to do with this process. Each month the young women struggle to deal with their periods; only a handful knew why and none would draw any conclusions were their periods absent. The 'big secret' is well served by these young women who, despite their own lack of understanding, conspire to keep the discomfort, tension, mess and pain hidden from the young men with whom they live—only one young man had some vague information about periods while thirty had none.

Other studies (see for example Katz 1974; Lowes 1977) confirm that the mentally handicapped as a group are isolated from clear information or support, but stress that they remain prey to the confused and exploiting messages of the media. Against this background many people, parents and staff alike, feel that it is better to 'say nothing and hope for the best', an attitude which leaves handicapped people bewildered and vulnerable.

Problem areas

The problems mentally handicapped people face in regard to their sexuality are a function of their own awareness and their involve-ment in the community.

Some of our students are grossly limited in both these respects and opportunities for exploration and independent experiences have been so limited that this complete lack of awareness is a problem in itself. Sadly some individuals, particularly those who are physically dependent, seem not to own their own bodies. Functions such as bowel movements are discussed and documented over their heads and they are often touched in a professional and impersonal way by carers. Their bodies may have been a source of pain or humiliation and without control over their bodily functions they may have no experience of privacy or consent. Games and exercises which restore the right of consent to them, at least in social situations, may help to restore a sense of dignity and establish their body as a source of sensation, pleasure, and expression.

Those who perceive themselves as fundamentally different because of physical deformity or handicap may not even identify with able-bodied adults and live in a limbo where there are no models on whom to base their expectations. Some may believe that they will get better as they grow older—a hope which is belied by their experience; or equally damagingly believe that because there are no adults like them, they will not grow up. Contact with older people who are themselves disabled and who are prepared to share the joys and limitations of their lifestyle is invaluable to them. I was often asked why there were no handicapped people in the slides I used to illustrate our discussions, and the underlying question "Are we like other people?" is one which recurs throughout our sessions.

For this group there is a powerful myth that sharing information will unleash desires and conflicts which will otherwise stay unawakened—a 'let sleeping dogs lie' approach. In fact the very opposite seems true because such ignorance is a lonely position to occupy without stress and a sense of being excluded is voiced by even our least assertive and articulate young people. To draw a veil over such basic matters as the processes at work in our bodies and the sexual attraction which is at the core of many adult relationships is to undermine their confidence in figuring out what is happening. As one young man explained, "My mam told me not to talk about it but I don't know what it is." These issues are likely to remain invisible within an institution and may even arise in response to the values inherent in our care system. Individuals thus characterised by their isolation are often those overlooked or screened out of any personal or sexual education which may be available and their lack of understanding used as a bar to situations in which it might be gained.

Impetus for a sex education programme will more often come from young people who need guidance about behaviour which is socially acceptable. We have a responsibility to set clear limits although the key concepts of privacy and consent are difficult to convey to those who may not have experienced either.

The issues are complicated by the fact that there are few norms agreed by all sections of society and it is helpful if staff can get together with parents to establish a consensus, even if it is a conservative one. Any guidelines are likely to be better than none.

There is also unease surrounding this whole area for us as members of a staff team whose colleagues may profoundly disagree with our stance and this insecurity renders us more likely to turn a blind eye or try to deal with inappropriate behaviour by distracting the person rather than confronting the issue. Masturbation is a simple example to draw on: our staff have decided in a meeting that masturbation should be regarded as acceptable within the privacy of the bedroom or toilets. Yet often this message is not conveyed to students with any clarity. We accept in other areas of social skills training that nuances and disapproving looks are ineffective and replacing them with direct instructions such as "No, John, don't pick your nose on the bus". A similar explicit instruction might be "Do not touch your penis when you are in the classroom". Our willingness to give this kind of clear instruction is tentative and while some of us are comfortable being clear in words, we may balk at showing someone where to masturbate, or pointing or gesturing to those who have difficulty understanding, especially the many deaf students we have whose language and communiciation skills are limited. Thus where there is ambivalence about the will, we do not always find a way.

Our failure to make clear the behaviour which is generally unacceptable pales by comparison with our unwillingness to give permission and express acceptance of sexual behaviour which *is* appropriate. Sexuality is always defined as a problem so that the issue we are discussing is essentially "What sexual behaviour is OK for people who are mentally handicapped". We do not deal with the issue of bad manners by persuading people not to eat.

Moral standards which rely on abstract thinking present problems to those whose simplicity renders them impervious to social conditioning and it is hard to justify our stance on issues such as homosexuality to them. Reduced to a level where such behaviour can be discussed in sign language the conversation might begin: "You are not bad, but you must not do it". This is a contradiction out of which the majority of us learn to be 'discreet' but the naiveté of mentally handicapped people remains to challenge the morals of us all.

A review of the incident book in a typical residential establishment might reveal the following 'problems'. It is useful to be aware of those feelings, attitudes and behaviours which cause distress to the individuals concerned and those which are defined as a problem by law or societal norms.

"Martin is masturbating in the TV room and is angry when he is told to go to his room."

"Patrick is found in the toilet with Jim; they have been masturbating together. He says it is Jim's fault and is so upset by the incident that he throws a temper tantrum."

"Sylvia and Garry are found together on the bed without their clothes on. When challenged and asked what they have been doing they are unable to explain. Both feel unhappy and ashamed after this exchange."

"Michael has been told that masturbating is sinful, he wants to know what it means."

"Katherine has a crush on one of the staff. She talks about him all day and the other students are nagging her about this until she loses her temper."

Documenting issues and incidents of this kind is a useful starting point and indicator of the kind of programme most needed. A simple analysis of problems into those concerned with knowing, doing or feeling helps to indicate the balance which should be achieved. Moreover such a record acts as a focus for gaining the support of colleagues, a support which is essential if you are to embark on a programme without ambiguity.

It is pertinent to remember the extreme examples of our failure to overcome confusion and inertia and make clear the options mentally handicapped people have in regard to their sexuality. Where they are in contact with the community the dangers *to them* of inappropriate sexual behaviour are out of proportion to the threat which they present to others.

Mentally handicapped people appearing before the courts for sex-related offences are characterised by their:

(1) Inability to mix with other adults, being unable to associate with others and consequently being either isolated or lonely individuals.

(2) Inability to understand a normal relationship; misinterpreting the friendliness of another person as an invitation to sexual relations.

(3) Susceptibility to influence by others, having been encouraged or introduced into sexual misconduct by other offenders.

135

(4) Lack of sexual knowledge, incomplete and distorted knowledge of sexual matters being directly related to the offences committed.

(5) Lack of control of impulses, exercising very little control over emotions and impulses (Cambridge Dept. of Criminal Science, 1957).

The plight of those who are hospitalised or imprisoned for acts deriving from ignorance, inadequacy or confusion represents a powerful argument for bringing sexuality into the mainstream of special education and training.

Mentally handicapped people do not live in isolation and even if they avoid for themselves the issues arising from sexual behaviour they may be confronted with the consequences of other people's sexual lives. Family issues such as divorce, the introduction of a new partner, the activities of siblings and so forth may be difficult to interpret without basic information and our students have often used the information they gained to make sense of the relationships around them. Moreover as Lindsay Lowes points out, the environment may itself be damaging:

> Communication between parents and siblings was often poor, families tending to be over protective and siblings themselves often being subjected to the pressures of unacceptable sexual habits within both their home and surrounding environments. Some trainees were exposed to incest or prostitution or exploited by a more experienced partner. (Lowes, 1977.)

Whether we are dealing with the growth of sexual identity, the development of appropriate behaviour or the sexual conduct of others, it is clear that our care for mentally handicapped people must include adequate information and support.

The social context of sex education

If a cool look at the problems is one factor in setting up a sensitive programme, another priority is to observe the relationships in the workplace between clients, staff and parents. Sexual behaviour and learning do not take place in isolation and are greatly affected by the quality of personal relationships available in an individual's day-to-day living situation. Lack of personal skills or self control, or the ability to express feelings, may well lead to problems of an overtly sexual nature, and the acquisition of appropriate and enjoyable social behaviour may be seen as a prerequisite to the development of appropriate sexual behaviour.

Young people entering Dene College at sixteen from residential special schools tend to be overly dependent on adults to the exclusion of and sometimes at the expense of their peers. They view each other as competition and since their programmes at school have often concentrated on individual teaching they frequently discount each other as a source of information, help or attention. The following incident illustrates this:

> Kenneth is sitting in the hall with twenty other students. He cannot talk but cries out to draw attention to the fact that he is slipping out of his wheelchair. None of the students respond, either by lifting him (of which several are capable) or by fetching a member of staff,

We therefore involve all our students in ongoing discussion groups of 6–8 people where we work to develop the peer group and to shift the emphasis from the staff as a resource to the group.

One such group, meeting for the first time, demonstrated their inability to relate to each other on any social level. The session was chaotic; they neither listened to, not looked at, each other. Concentration varied and individuals left the group at will.

Initially we set the ground rules for our session.

This group agreed to be bounded by the following agreement:

(1) We meet on Tuesday afternoon from 1.30–3.00 p.m.

(2) We will not all talk at once, we will take turns.

(3) Everyone will wait while the teacher signs to Robert.

(4) No burping or singing in our sessions.

(5) We will take no notice when Andy acts silly.

Over the next five or six weeks these rules need to be consistently brought to their attention. We share information about our homes and families, our schools, our involvement in the College. Two students go to youth club so we practise in role play being new in such a situation. We discuss different handicaps ensuring that those who are handicapped by deafness or communication problems are given appropriate consideration. My role in the group at this stage is highly directive; I assert the rules, formally give each person their say, and deal with any problem behaviour explaining to the group what I am doing, for example:

> I do not want to give Andy any time for burping—so I am going to ignore him until he acts sensibly again.

Six weeks later we conclude a session in which everyone has played a part. The students noticed that we had observed our rules and that the discussion had been orderly.

This initial process of group building will vary according to the different contexts in which we work. Where there is a natural peer group for example in a ward, or group home, a regular period of time set aside for consideration of relationships, achievements and problems, will hasten this. Such a forum is ideal as a place for the sharing of information on sexuality.

Sharing information about sexuality

The following teaching notes suggest an outline of areas which we aim to cover.

Each group, however, determines the order in which the information is presented and the amount of time devoted to each topic. I do not have a syllabus in mind, with a certain amount of information to be presented in each session, lest I miss cues from individuals about what is important for them. Flexible resources, visual aids and so forth, enable us to return to areas which have been forgotten or move on to new ground when we are ready.

In each area there are three levels on which to work. Firstly we are responsive to the feelings which are expressed whether they be guilt or sadness, caring or frustration because the group may be the only place in which such feelings can be explored. Secondly, we use clear language and explicit pictures and slides to convey the basic facts of life, adapting our approach to differing levels of understanding and specific disabilities such as deafness or communication difficulties. Thirdly, we help these young people make decisions about their sexual options bearing in mind the morals they have imbibed from parents and others and their own growing awareness of the issues involved. Together we set guidelines for behaviour within our own community.

1. We establish the group as a place where we can talk openly about sex and make a contract about what we are going to do on the lines of:

> We do not usually talk about sex because it is private, but we are going to make a special agreement to talk about it here because it is important for you to know about growing up. Is that OK with you?

This leads into a discussion of previous sex education, at home or school and the feelings of embarrassment which may surround it.

I do not feel that it is necessary to assess in detail the knowledge of the group at this stage, although there are several excellent tools which can be used for this purpose (see for example Davies, 1980). Because we do not stream or screen out individuals in this programme each group contains people operating at different levels whose needs vary from the simplest of immediate information to the consideration of complex issues. Thus the ethos is of the group pooling its knowledge and feelings and each individual taking what is appropriate to his needs from the whole.

2. Our goal is to establish each person as a young man or woman, firstly by dealing with the distinction between male and female, and secondly by asserting that the students are now young adults rather than children.

We draw together different terms for men and women, including signs and symbols. Using games we distinguish between male and female christian names and look at relationships such as mother and father, and son and daughter. Conferring adult status is an important element in our groups. We talk about growing up, using pictures of young people at different stages of development and deciding when boys and girls become men and women. We role play situations in which we introduce each other as Mr. Smith and Miss Lewis—a status which mentally handicapped people are rarely afforded.

3. The difference between men and women are explored, beginning with the more social ones such as beards, different hair-styles, clothes and so forth. Then when the group is comfortable we use slides of naked men and women to point out the basic physical differences. We seek to establish a comfortable style and terminology at this point collecting together different terms current in the group for the sexual organs and agreeing on the names we will use.

4. We concentrate on men's bodies and how they work, including erections, semen and sperm, and wet dreams.

5. We consider how women's bodies work in regard both to the reasons for and management of periods and show examples of different kinds of sanitary protection.

6. Masturbation is a central issue and in addition to basic information about how and why both men and women masturbate we establish, often by walking round the College, which areas are private and public. We talk about sexy feelings, crushes and day-dreams, accepting each other's fantasies and feelings.

139

7.   Adult relationships need to be deciphered and some norms agreed on how to behave at different stages of a relationship. We talk to people around the College about their boyfriends and girlfriends, how long they have been married and so forth, bringing together the information into some coherent guidelines about the commitments and sexual content of these relationships.

Such norms are bound to be somewhat contrived but they act as the basis for acceptable behaviour within the day-to-day living situation and as protection for those who are not able to interpret subtle messages indicating consent.

8.   Intercourse is explained within the context of loving relationships and where it is appropriate we discuss positions which are useful for disabled people and even the possibility of future help being available in residential establishments.

The nature of consent is essential to convey and some information about rape and its seriousness included.

9.   Individual counselling is given to anyone who is considered in need of contraceptive advice but the methods and advantages of each are discussed with those whose need is not urgent but for whom it is important to establish that marriage and parenthood are separate issues.

10.   Where babies really come from! Here we discuss the growth of the fetus using models and a film which culminates in a birth. Pregnant friends are drafted in and cross-examined.

11.   The responsibilities of parenthood and childcare are considered and we assess each other's abilities and disabilities in reference to the needs of children.

12.   Homosexuality needs to be accepted as a part of growing up although sadly the legal implications force us to limit such expression as none of the students are over twenty-one years old.

Outcomes

The emotional aura which so often surrounds sex education can lead both teachers and students beforehand to magnify and blow up the subject out of all proportion. In our experience, working with these groups of young handicapped people, what actually happens is a deflating, yet at the same time an enhancing process. What starts out with some embarrassment, as a big deal, is often seen as 'obvious' when we have finished and the students forget that they were ever in the dark. Nevertheless they wear such awareness like a badge. A knowledge of basic facts brings a sense of relief which allows many of them to move on to deal sensibly and maturely with personal issues and decisions which arise from their sharing of the 'secret'.

A prime response to this information is often at the level of helping individuals to understand their own position in the world. Discussion on birth and the development of the fetus most often revolve around our own development, rather than the implications of parenthood. This emerges as a fundamental gap in these young people's self knowledge. We spend some time on variations of this theme using drawings and pictures both for illustration and to enable students to express their new understanding (see illustrations).

A further issue which is critical to our students is why and how some babies are born handicapped. Along with sex, this is a taboo subject and often no one has ever talked to, or even in front of, these multiply handicapped young people about the origins, or nature or prognosis of their handicap. Thus our discussions about being men and women are interlaced with the realisation of handicap and its implications. I assert the same values, especially honesty, in regard to this as to sexual issues. Exchanges like the following one have taught me not to underestimate people's ability to deal with the realities of their situation, when confronted kindly and honestly.

Alice: "My dad says I can get married when my arm gets better."
H.B.: "I don't think your arm will get better, Alice; what do you think?"
Alice: "Well, I don't think it will, either—it has been like this since I was born. My dad said he didn't want me to come out of hospital if I was handicapped; I heard him tell my mum that."

Another result of removing the barriers is that we can actively give young people permission to think about what is happening around them and make sense of the relationships they see as well as those in which they are involved. One group were discussing marriage in a sugary 'happy ever after' manner but when invited to look at each person within the group and their family experience the picture was different. One person was in care, and another had recently lost his mother; two students had divorced parents whose separation caused them some problems and two were from families who shared both joy and friction. None of this was new information; what we did was to use again the experiences we had shared to test an assumption freshly, in other words to practise thinking.

Woman   Baby   Man

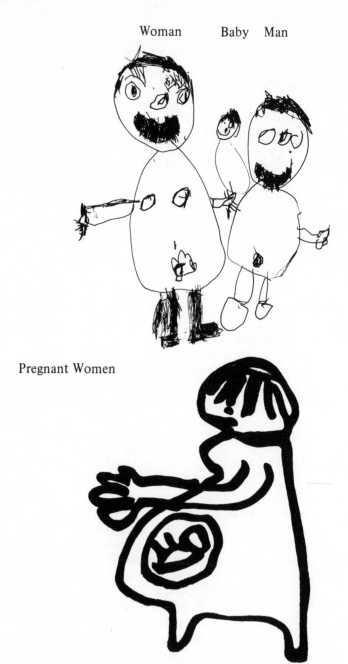

Pregnant Women

Reproduced by kind permission of the students, Ian and Trevor.

142

Increasing confidence in their ability to understand and work things out is a by-product of a programme which invites people to think in this way.

An issue in which this understanding was put to good use was that of parenthood. Many of these young people, whose physical as well as intellectual handicaps had led others to write-off their chances of parenthood were able to take their own look at the reasons. My fears in opening up the subject were that their conclusions would be irresponsible and unrealistic but this was not so. A severely physically handicapped young woman who had been told she could not have children, said she now realised that this was because she would not be able to look after a child. This made sense to her in a way that the general interdiction had not; it had become her choice and her decision. Another faced the physical problems which would prevent her undergoing a pregnancy with a frankness I had not envisaged, and while there were some sad feelings around this issue they were largely resolved.

What of the least able of our students whose intellectual handicaps made this 'progression' impossible? Is it worth including them in such a programme? Our study showed that those with mental ages recorded at three years or under were unable to grasp any but the most immediate information, but I believe that these groups are a valid forum in which to convey even that. Peer group pressure is valuable in modifying behaviour and it makes sense to give explicit instructions, for example about masturbation, in a group of this kind. Thus, as group leader, I have different goals and expectations for individual members of the group. Success for one young man whom I had consistently asked not to masturbate in our sessions came when he retorted:

"I am going to sit in the bathroom for hours when I get out of here!"

Another significant outcome was improved peer group relationships. I discovered the possibility of working on social development and sex education inadvertently. My first venture with a group formed specifically to impart basic sexual information failed because we tackled delicate matters 'cold'. Learning from this I prepared future groups carefully, not moving into discussions about sexuality until they were comfortable with me and with each other. I was in turn surprised and moved by the effect of our session on relationships within the group. Having worked through our embarrassment, the sharing of sexual information and private feelings galvanised the group and led us on to franker and more mature discussions on other issues.

This experience is confirmed by Lindsey Lowes (1977), describing the follow-up to a sex education programme in an Adult Training Centre:

> On completion and at the trainees' own request integrated sessions have developed on a weekly basis when the trainees are able to discuss sexual, emotional, psychological or other problems.

This strongly suggests that mentally handicapped young people make good use of a regular opportunity to discuss with each other, their feelings and relationship. Such a forum can be used to deal with problem behaviour, to initiate schemes and activities and to promote understanding of other people. Managers and teachers will know how much time and energy go into such matters and yet an ad hoc approach dissipates our efforts and minimises the opportunities which exist to learn from the experience of others.

The picture in Adult Training Centres

Faced with ambivalence from staff and parents the picture which emerges in Adult Training Centres is that the majority of sexual incidents are discussed on an individual ad hoc basis. This usually implies that such counselling as is available is in response to 'trouble', when lack of basic sexual knowledge can compound the problem. For example John and Mary are found together in a state of undress and it is important for us to know if intercourse has taken place. This is not the time for a sex education lesson but the question "Did he put his penis inside you" can be put calmly and if the answer is "Yes", gives those of us responsible in such situations the information we need.

Staff in training centres are not able to proceed in this way where they are anxious about the response of the authorities or of parents, and discussions about such a programme as well as the responsibilities involved in setting appropriate limits make possible a more relaxed and constructive approach to a whole range of personal relationships.

The London Borough of Greenwich is one among several authorities who moved in this direction by holding two-day conferences for parents and staff involved in their centres. The days included a presentation on the needs for a programme and slides which might be used with ample time for discussion in small groups.

Many parents who began by fearing such a programme were able to see that it might help them. Their anxiety focussed on the possibility of upsetting the delicate balance they had achieved. Many did not limit themselves to discussing sexual issues but welcomed an opportunity to share difficulties, such as those of bereavement, which they had borne alone. The burden of caring for mentally handicapped people has fallen largely on parents whose lives are dogged with the uncertainty of "What will happen when we die?" We pay lip service to the 'normalisation' of life styles for mentally handicapped people but their parents also need this consideration. Parents justifiably resent being told how they should approach sensitive issues when they feel that they might in the long run 'be left holding the baby'. According mentally handicapped people the respect and dignity due to them as adults is a process in which sex education plays a small, if important, part. As many parents reiterated throughout these discussions the need for a range of residential facilities within the community is a priority. Meanwhile parents need access to self-help groups and professional support services which will ease their loneliness and enable them to work together demanding relevant services.

Conclusion

In keeping young people ignorant about sex, and about the nature of their handicaps, we cannot maintain the pretence that we are doing nothing. In fact we achieve such an end by lying and discounting, by ignoring feelings which are important to the people to whom we are responsible and by repressing behaviour which we find difficult to channel into appropriate relationships. To be on the receiving end of such dismissal is not comfortable; as one young man replied when asked what he felt about being kept in the dark:

"It's not just wrong, it's rotten."

In giving information about sexuality we are not abdicating responsibility but opening the possibility of sharing it with young people whose ability to take decisions will vary as much as the situations they encounter. Even where our judgement leads us to step in we owe it to those in our care that we decide vital issues with them and not for them. A sensitive programme of sex education establishes mentally handicapped young people as adults in our

145

community and challenges us to provide services which are worthy of that status.

REFERENCES

Brown, H. (1980). Sexual Knowledge and Education of ESN Students in Centers of Education. *Sexuality and Disability 3*, 3, 215–20.
Cambridge Department of Criminal Science (1957). *Sexual Offences*. London: Macmillan.
Davies, M (1980). *Sex Education for Slow Learners: A Teaching Aid*. SPOD, The Diorama, 14 Peto Place, London NW1 4DT.
Katz, G. (1974). Sex Education for Mentally Retarded Adults in Sweden. In: Lee, G., and Katz, G. *The Sexual Rights of the Retarded*. London: NSMHC.
Lowes, L. (1977). *Sex and Social Training*. London: NSMHC.

CHAPTER 8

A Health and Sex Education Programme: Curriculum and Resources

Ann Craft, * *Jean Davis, Maldwyn Williams and Marjorie Williams*

Any curriculum is an outline, and an outline has to be filled in by the people using it. Many may consider this an overinclusive programme, but it is intended to suggest a structure which may be adapted according to age, need and circumstance.

It evolved in the setting of a mental handicap hospital, and was primarily designed for those adolescent and adult residents who are potentially capable of living in the community, either independently or in sheltered housing. It has taken a year to work through the programme, with sessions most weeks which last for about an hour, this including a cup of tea and biscuits. We have been flexible as to the order of some of the topics, following interests that arose, or returning to subjects to refresh our knowledge. For example, one group moved from learning about conception and pregnancy under "The Human Body" module, to thinking about the demands of parenthood and methods of contraception. We returned again to these topics in the context of "Adulthood". Some groups omitted certain topics completely, exploring others in great detail.

A variety of teaching strategies have been used: role play and 'pretend' situations; making charts and posters; and practical competitions such as spotting the number of hazards 'planted' in our kitchen.

We have tried to always link examples to events and circumstances in the lives of the individuals in the group, and help them to share their experiences.

Use of Audiovisual Resources

Having something to look at and to speak to can be an enormous help in learning and teaching. It gives a focus to a discussion, and

* Ann Craft would like to thank the Marie Stopes Research Fund whose grant enabled her to undertake counselling sessions and to hire or purchase audiovisual resources for use in the programme.

can be a means for both teacher* and students to avoid embarrassment. Even something as simple as pictures cut from a magazine can provide that extra stimulus which makes the difference between a topic being remembered or forgotten.

Books, pictures, slides, filmstrips and videotapes are all flexible to use—the teacher can pick out what is suitable for any particular mentally handicapped individual or group. Films do not allow you to stop and explain or get comments about a particular point, but they have a place in any health and sex education programme, and the teacher can make a note of discussion points to take up afterwards.

Your local Health Education Officer and/or the Education Officer concerned with Special Schools may be able to arrange for you to borrow audiovisual material and equipment. There may be an educational resource centre in your area which lends out films, etc. There is one caveat which teachers should bear in mind—the majority of resources are not specifically designed for a mentally handicapped audience. Care and sensitivity is needed for instance, when using material designed for normal children, with mentally handicapped adults. Body models and skeletons are fun to use when talking about the way the human body works. Your local hospital or Nurse Training School may allow you to borrow or visit and look at their teaching models. Pictures from magazines can illustrate different foods, expressions, people, races, sexes and behaviour. Someone who draws well could illustrate a set of 'moral dilemma' situations, eg, accepting a lift in a car; seeing a shoplifter at work; a man's hand on the knee of a woman beside him on the bus. Your local newspaper will give or sell cheaply, end-of-the-roll paper which can be either cut up for project books, or used to show people's height and outline. With a little imagination you can compile your own resources file.

We have indicated some of the audiovisual material available against each topic, but this is not exhaustive, and the reader is advised to obtain a copy of the Review of Resources published by the Health Education Council.†

* We use the term 'teacher' loosely, meaning simply the person who is presenting the topic and leading the discussion.

†Craft, A. (1982). *Health, Hygiene and Sex Education for Mentally Handicapped Children, Adolescents and Adults: A Review of Audio-visual Resources*. Available free from The Resources Centre, Health Education Council, 71-75 New Oxford Street, London WC1A 1AH.

The Human Body

This may seem to be too detailed, indeed many of us have only a sketchy knowledge about the location of our internal organs, and the job they do, yet manage to live our lives quite satisfactorily. But we have opened our curriculum with several units concerned with the workings of the human body not with the intention of a crash course on biology, but to allow people to talk about their bodies in a context and atmosphere very different from those usually pertaining. As mentally handicapped children grow up the majority come to see their bodies as somehow 'dirty', something to make jokes and giggle about. Not that there won't be giggles, sniggers and jokes in the group, but the leaders must show by their attitude and matter-of-fact approach that bodies and the way they work can indeed be funny and jokeworthy, but certainly not 'dirty'.

A very basic knowledge does give a foundation to which we can link most of the other topics—good health, hygiene, physical development, safety, etc. and the visit to the Nurse Training School's skeleton and body model has remained in the students' memories.

THE HUMAN BODY

Topic	Approach
THE SKELETON	

1. Why do we have a skeleton?
    framework for support
    protection
    joints
    what happens when bones break?
	(a) Feeling our bones and moving different kinds of joints
	(b) Body models and skeleton
	(c) Games naming parts of the body

2. How do bones move? muscles and tendons	

3. Skin covers skeletons
    it is waterproof
    sensitive
    regulates body temperature by pores	

THE HUMAN BODY

Topic	Approach
INSIDE OUR BODIES	
1. The heart 　　what it looks like 　　what it does 2. The lungs 　　what they look like 　　what they do 　　good breathing 3. Blood circulation 　　what is blood for? 　　arteries and veins 　　blood transfusions and donors 4. The brain 　　what it does 　　brain damage, eg loss of 　　　memory, stroke 5. The nervous system 　　sensory (feeling pain, etc.) 　　motor (controlling movement)	(a) Feel your heart beating, 　　listen with stethoscope (b) Feel your pulse (c) Deep breathing, fill your lungs (d) Relaxation techniques to get 　　us in touch with our bodies, 　　e.g. blowing up imaginary 　　balloons, tie the top, find a 　　pin and 1—2—3 BANG! 　　Divide into pairs, one blowing 　　the other up as a balloon 　　(expanding from curled, 　　crouched position on floor 　　until standing fat and tall). 　　Burst with imaginary pin. 　　"Balloon" collapses. (e) Likening the brain and 　　nervous system to the HQ of 　　an army, with messages 　　coming and going from 　　outlying companies.
Topic	*Approach*
WHAT HAPPENS TO THE FOOD WE EAT	
1. Mouth 　　tongue tastes 　　teeth chew 　　saliva moistens 　　throat swallows 2. Stomach 　　gastric juices 　　digestion begins 3. Intestines 　　digestion continues 　　food absorbed into body 4. Elimination 　　waste material to bowels— 　　　leaves body via anus 　　other waste dissolved by kid- 　　　neys, becomes urine, leaves 　　　body via bladder and urethra.	(a) The small and large intestines 　　together measure about 　　22 feet. Measure this out with 　　a cord or rope, then try to 　　coil it as small as possible.

Topic	Approach
THE SENSES	
1. Sight—eyes 　what is seeing? 　blindness 2. Smell—nose 　what is smelling? 　imagine you can't smell 3. Touch—nerves and fingers 　what does touch tell us? 4. Hearing—ears 　how do we hear? 　deafness 5. Taste—tongue 　is taste important? 　what if you couldn't taste 　　anything you ate?	(a) Simple experiments using a blindfold, identifying and describing different objects and textures by touch; different foods by taste; different odours by smell; telling where sound in a room comes from by hearing alone. (b) Games such as: 　(i) one person blindfolded in middle of a circle. Circle moves round and stops. Blindfolded person touches someone and has to tell who it is by gently feeling. 　(ii) Divide into two lines and pair with opposite person. Each pair selects an animal noise. Everyone closes eyes, lines reshuffled. Find partner by making agreed animal noise.

Topic	Approach
REPRODUCTIVE SYSTEMS	
1. Male and female reproductive systems 2. How a human baby is made 3. Pregnancy 4. Different reproductive systems, eg birds, cats, fish.	(a) Visit by a woman who is pregnant perhaps at monthly intervals so that the group can ask questions and see the pregnancy progress. (b) Encourage students to look at themselves in a full-length mirror when next they have a bath, and to use a small hand mirror to look at their genital area.

REFERENCES: THE HUMAN BODY

BOOKS

Althea (1975). *A Baby In The Family*. Cambridge: Dinosaur Publications.
Andry, A.C. and Schepp, S. (1969). *How Babies Are Made*. London: Time-Life International.
Chovil, C. and Jones, E.G. (1977). *How Did I Grow?* London: BBC Publications.
Clark, P.M. and Burgess, J. (eds.) (1979). *You And Your Body*. London: Macmillan.
Daniel, D.S. (1967). *Your Body*. Loughborough: Ladybird Books. (Also available as a 25-frame colour film strip.)
Elkington, T. and Ward, J. (1979). *Biology You Need*. Sunbury-on-Thames: Nelson.
Fagerstrom, G. and Hansson, G. (1979). *Our New Baby*. London: Macdonald Educational.
Halford, S. (1978). *Teeth*. Loughborough: Ladybird Books. (Also available as a colour film strip.)
Howard, J. (1978). *The Human Body*. London: Macdonald Educational.
Johnson, V. and Williams, T. (1979). *Good Health*. Book 1. Sunbury-on-Thames: Nelson.
Mayle, P. (1978). *Where Did I Come From?* London: Macmillan.
Moyle, D. (ed.) (1975). *The Human Body*. London: Macdonald Educational. Easy Reading Edition.
Nilsson, L. (1975). *How You Began*. Harmondsworth: Kestrel Books.
Rayner, C. (1978). *The Body Book*. London: G. Whizzard/Andre Deutsch.
Schools Council Project (1977). *How Did I Begin?* Unit 2 of "All About Me" series. Sunbury-on-Thames: Nelson.
Sheffield, M. (1973). *Where Do Babies Come From?* London: Jonathan Cape. (Education Resource Centres may have a copy of the BBC radiovision filmstrip based on the book. It is now no longer available for purchase.)
Spiers, H. (1971). *How You Began*. J.M. Dent & Sons.

FILMS, SLIDES, VIDEO (for addresses of distributors see page 185)

Discovering Your Senses
  Your Eyes are for Seeing
  Your Ears are for Hearing
  Your Skin is for Feeling
  Your Tongue is for Tasting
  Your Nose is for Smelling
  Your Senses Work Together
	Pack of six American film strips, cassettes, and teachers' notes.
	View Tech Audiovisual Media

The Five Senses
  Hearing
  Sight
  Touch
  Smell
  Taste
	Four slide sets of 12 slides with teachers' notes.
	The Slide Centre

How Babies are Born	16mm colour 10 min film. Eothen Films International Limited.
Inside the Body	32-frame colour film strip, cassette and teachers' notes, BBC Publications

153

Merry-go-round	BBC television programme.
1. Beginning	BBC Enterprises *or* Videorecord off air
2. Birth	
3. Full Circle	
Sexuality and the Mentally Handicapped	Set of Winifred Kempton's teaching slides.
I Parts of the body	Available for hire from FPA *or* SPOD;
V Human Reproduction	Purchase from Concord Films *or*
	E. Patterson Assoc. Limited

MISCELLANEOUS

Body Parts Dice Game. Playing Board (30 × 40 cm). Taskmaster.
Digesting Our Food. Large Chart (76 × 100 cm). Pictorial Charts.

Good Health

This section may well provoke questions and discussion, not only from the mentally handicapped students, but also from the staff of school, ATC, hostel or hospital. It is an appropriate point to review the opportunities available to students, residents or trainees, for example what possibilities are there for healthy exercise? Starting a voluntary 'keep fit' class could be one way to encourage people to exercise more. Many mentally handicapped people have a degree of physical handicap, and your local physiotherapy department should be able to help you devise a series of simple exercises, including one or two for those in wheelchairs. Again, it is of little use exhorting students to watch the kind of food they eat when they have little or no choice of main meals, and fruit is not nearly so available as sweets and chocolate. *If we do not provide, perhaps create, opportunities for students to put principles into practice, we are wasting our time and theirs.*

GOOD HEALTH

Topic	Approach
FOOD, DIET & EATING HABITS	

1. Why do we eat?
  to make our bodies strong
    and grow
  warmth and energy
  help body fight disease
  we eat *TO LIVE*
	(a) Body needs fuel, like a car
	(b) Make individual charts of
	  different types of food with
	  magazine pictures

2. Our bodies need
  PROTEIN
  CARBOHYDRATE
  FAT
  VITAMINS
  ROUGHAGE
	(c) Get students to record
	  everything eaten and drunk
	  for one day (staff or parents
	  to help if necessary).

3. Balancing our food intake
  danger of 'junk' foods
	(d) Keep individual weight charts
	  over several weeks.

4. Importance of liquid intake
  helps our kidneys work well
  dehydration
	(e) Plan and discuss a menu for
	  a week.
	  (Incidentally, do students
	  understand what is meant by
	  dishes such as shepherd's pie
	  or Welsh rarebit?)

5. Dangers of overeating and
  overweight
    shortness of breath
    varicose veins
    foot trouble
    backache
    high blood pressure
    diabetes
    stroke
    heart attack	

Topic	Approaches
EXERCISE, GOOD BREATHING, SLEEP	

1. What is exercise?
    making our bodies work,
    especially our muscles
2. Why should we exercise?
    improves our bodies
    helps reduce tension
    keeps weight down
    improves circulation
    helps muscles grow
3. Dangers of not exercising
    obesity
    sluggishness
4. How should we exercise?
5. Deep, not shallow breathing to get more
    OXYGEN into lungs, more
    CARBON DIOXIDE out
6. Importance of sleep to body
    individual variations of need
	(a) In pairs, measure pulse rate, breathing rate and temperature after five minutes vigorous exercise
	(b) Examples of simple body exercises
	(c) Deep breathing exercises
	(d) Make a chart of amount and type of exercise taken during one week
	(e) Keep a chart for a week of the time you went to bed and the time you got up

Topic	Approaches
SAFETY OF SELF AND OTHERS	

1. What causes accidents?
    carlessness
    familiarity
    human error/misjudgment
2. What should we do in emergencies?
    simple first aid
    fire
3. Accidents are one of the major causes of death
    home—falls, poisons, cuts, electric, burns
    road—safety drills
    industrial—tools
4. Signs of illness—what do we do?
    role of the doctor
        and specialist
    going to hospital
5. Safe travel
    bus
    car
    pedestrian
	(a) Demonstration of simple first aid, eg cuts, fainting, epileptic fit
	(b) Short talk by local Fire Officer
	(c) Set up a room with hazards, how many are spotted?
	(d) Make a list of common symptoms of illness, eg pain, nausea, discharges, fever
	(e) Role play describing symptoms of an illness to a nurse or doctor
	(f) List the potentially dangerous areas in the locality. What precautions should we take for each?

GOOD HEALTH

Topic	Approaches
SMOKING	
1. What happens to our bodies when we smoke?	(a) Get a smoker to exhale while smoking through a paper tissue to show nicotine stain left
2. What makes people take their first cigarette?	
3. "Advantages" of smoking being one of the crowd (grown-up) calms you—relieves tension	(b) Collect different cigarette advertisements—what do they seem to promise?
4. Disadvantages of smoking cancer coughs, bronchitis heart disease damage of lungs cost nicotine stains breath smells	(c) Count up the financial cost per week, per month, per year, to smokers in the group (d) Aids to cut down or stop smoking, such as nicotine gum (e) Use a magnifying glass on paper to show how easily broken glass can start a fire
5. Danger smoking in bed cigarette end in wastepaper bin obeying "No Smoking" signs eg petrol stations, trains, restaurants starting fires in countryside	
6. Cutting down or stopping smoking? can we do it?	

Topic	Approaches
DRUGS	
1. Purpose of drugs to cure or prevent illness; relieve pain; cure disease; ease tension	(a) Make a list of common instructions, eg Do not exceed the stated dose; Not suitable for children; take one tablet three times a day What do these mean?
2. Dangers of drugs side effects incorrect dose taking someone else's drugs with alcohol	(b) Role play—what to do if someone offers you "a pill to make you happy"
3. Dangers of "glue-sniffing"	

Topic	Approaches
ALCOHOL	

1. What is alcohol?
    a food or a drug
    name different drinks with
        various alcohol levels
	(a) Role playing, how we might
	        refuse a drink

2. Why do people drink?
    recreation—pub, social
        occasion
    relaxes
    with meals
    makes them cheerful (for a
        time only);
    habit
    mental escape from unpleasant
        or upsetting situation
	(b) Role play a drunk in a group;
	        what trouble does he/she
	        cause?
	(c) Collect magazine advertise-
	        ments and refer to TV com-
	        mercials. What do they
	        promise?
	(d) Set up a courtroom situa-
	        tion—a drunken driver or a
	        drunken pedestrian has
	        caused a serious accident.
	        What penalty should be
	        imposed?

3. Effect on body
    varies with height or weight,
        amount of food in stomach,
        emotional state
    distorts perception and speed
        of response
    affects nerves controlling
        movement.	

4. Dangers of alcohol
    loss of self-control and false
        sense of well-being
    makes you careless and
        clumsy—accidents
    vomiting
    hangover
    sad
    loss of appetite
    addiction
    liver damage—shrinks and
        hardens
    brain damage—poisons cells
    liability to friends
    aggression	

5. Medication and alcohol	

6. Legal aspects
    age
    licensing laws
    offences and penalties	

Topic	Approaches
HANDICAPS	
1. What is a handicap?	(a) How many handicaps can the group list?
2. Handicaps of the senses, eg blindness. Handicaps of motor activity	(b) Spend 5 or 10 minutes pretending to be blind, deaf, paralysed, etc.
3. Nearly everyone has a handicap of one sort or another. These tend to increase with age	
4. How can we minimise (make less important) them? corrective devices (drugs for epilepsy, spectacles, hearing aids) accepting our handicaps but not letting them dominate our lives guarding against self pity	
5. Handicaps are as handicapping as we allow them to be	

REFERENCES: GOOD HEALTH

BOOKS

Baldwin, D. (1978). *Human Biology and Health*. London: Longman.

Health Education Council (1979). *Looking After Yourself!* Free booklet.

Health Education Council (1979). *The Smoker's Guide to Non-Smoking*. Free booklet.

Johnson, V. and Williams, T. (1979 and 1980). *Good Health*. Books 1 and 2. Sunbury-on-Thames: Nelson.

Latto, K. (1981). *Give Us the Chance. Sport and physical recreation with mentally handicapped people*. London: Disabled Living Foundation.

Matson, J.L. (1980). Preventing home accidents: a training program for the retarded. *Behavior modification, 4*, 3, 397–410.

Schools Council Project (1977). *What Helps Me Grow* and *Looking After Myself*. Units 4 and 5 of "All About Me" series. *From Sickness to Health, Deadly Decisions, Time to Spare, Food for Thought*, and *Skills and Spills*. Units 3, 4, 5, 6 and 8 of "Think Well" series. Sunbury-on-Thames: Nelson.

Smith, T., and Breckon, B. (1978). *Accident Action*. London: Macmillan.

Taylor, P. and Robinson, P. (1979). *Crossing the Road*. Kidderminster: British Institute of Mental Handicap publications.

159

GOOD HEALTH

FILMS, SLIDES, VIDEO (for addresses of distributors see page 185)

Accidents Don't Just Happen— *They Are Caused*	30 frame film strip, part (v) "Live and Learn" Series. Camera Talks Limited.
Educating Mentally Handicapped People	Camera Talks.
2. The Picture of Health	51 slides or film strip.
4. Watch Out in the Kitchen	44 slides or film strip.
5. This House is Dangerous	47 slides or film strip.
6. Look Out	49 slides or film strip.
Good Health	15-minute videos or 16 mm films of a
2. White Ivory	TV series.
3. Doctor Sweet-Tooth (previous title:	Central TV (formerly ATV) *or* Rank
The Good Food Programme)	Film Library.
4. Love Your Lungs	
5. Germs, Germs, Germs	
6. Watch Out!	
7. Fit and Healthy (previous title:	
Exercise and Rest)	
8. Talking Feet	
9. Time to Spare? (previous title:	
Fun and Games)	
13. Nurse!	
Good Health Habits	A set of 6 film strips with cassette
Keeping Well	commentary. View Tech Audiovisual
Keeping Clean	Media.
Your Food	
Your Clothes	
Your Rest and Sleep	
Good Health for You	37 frame film strip. Camera Talks.
The Healthy Way in Wonderland	American film strips, cassettes and
Miss Huff 'n' Puff's Exercise Troupe	teachers' notes. The Slide Centre.
Chef Ahmalette's Health Diet	
Let's Go—and Keep Fit	20-minute video or film of the BBC
and Cross the Road	programme. Record off air *or* Concord Films.
Spot The Hazard	29 slides or film strip. Camera Talks.
What Do You Think About Smoking?	33 slides or film strip. Camera Talks.
Where There's Smoke	16 mm 14-minute Canadian colour film. Concord Films.

MISCELLANEOUS

Goal: Beginning Health and Nutrition	82 lesson cards. Learning Development Aids.
Look After Yourself! and *Eat More Fresh* *Fruit and Vegetables!*	Large and colourful posters. Health Educational Council.
Playing the Health Game	Large chart (76 × 100 cm) designed as a board for a dice game. Pictorial Charts.
Project Fire	Home Office fire prevention pack. Teacher's notes, wall charts, project sheets. HMSO.
Taking the Strain	BBC LP record: REC407 or cassette: ZCM407.

160

Personal Hygiene

This module on 'Personal Hygiene', as the previous one on 'Good Health', should lead care-givers to re-appraise the living circumstances of the mentally handicapped students and their existing opportunities for personal decisions. It is relatively common to hear a comment such as "It's all very well to tell them to have a bath or a shower every day, but it's not just practical". Problems of supervision, a limited supply of fresh towels, availability of clean clothes, and the inflexibility of the 'bath book' may all combine to frustrate the mentally handicapped individual who wants a bath over and above his quota of two a week. Care of one's own body is made up of separate components, 'bricks' that go towards building up the total social skill of the student and as a welcome by-product, reduces the load on the care givers.

PERSONAL HYGIENE

Topic	*Approaches*
KEEPING CLEAN	

1. Why do we wash ourselves?
   to get rid of germs
   to get rid of sweat
   to get rid of dead skin
   to get rid of dirt
   to make sure we don't smell
	(a) List the things you need when
	     when taking a bath
	(b) Take off shoes—how smelly
	     are your feet? What about
	     other parts of your body, such
	     as armpits?

2. How often do we wash?
   our hands before meals,
     after toilet, before preparing
     and eating food
   when we get up and go to bed
   when we are dirty	

3. How often do we shower or
  bathe?
   at *least* once a week, more if
     we need it or feel like it	

4. On the days you don't bathe or
  shower, where should you wash?
   hands, face and neck
   genitals
   feet
   under arms	

5. Deodorants	

Topic	Approaches
GOOD GROOMING	

1. Care of hair?
    how often do we wash our hair?
    type of shampoo
    rinsing well
    washing comb and brushes
    Head lice ("nits")
2. Fingernails
    cutting or filing
    nailbrush
    getting dirt out
    use of nail varnish and remover
    hang-nails
    biting nails
3. Make-up for girls
    for different occasions
    importance of cleansing skin
    importance of moisturiser
4. General appearance
    neatness
    cleanliness of self and clothes
	(a) Imagine you are going out somewhere special; how would you get yourself ready?
	(b) Make-up demonstration
	(c) Ways of stopping nail-biting
	(d) Polishing shoes
	(e) Using a clothes brush
	(f) Sewing on buttons

Topic	Approaches
CHANGING OUR CLOTHES	

1. How often should we change our:
    underclothes
    socks/tights
    shirts/blouses
    trousers/skirts
2. If we wash our clothes by hand, what parts of them need special attention:
    cuffs
    under arms
    crotch
3. Care of clothes:
    hanging them up
    folding neatly
	(a) Demonstration of washing underclothes, tights, socks;
	(b) Demonstrate hanging up clothes: folding them neatly in drawers.

PERSONAL HYGIENE

Topic	Approaches
CARE AND CLEANING OF TEETH	

1. Purpose of teeth
  cut and slice food (incisors canines)
2. How many sets do we have?
  baby (milk)
  permanent
3. Keeping our teeth clean and healthy
  how do we brush them?
  foods which are bad for teeth
  plaque and decay
  good toothbrush, fluoride paste
4. False teeth
	(a) Arrange visit from Dental Hygiene Officer
	(b) Use disclosing tablets to show plaque left on teeth
	(c) Care of false teeth

Topic	Approaches
MENSTRUAL HYGIENE FOR FEMALES	

1. Importance of:
  wearing sanitary pads or tampons
  changing them as needed
  taking last tampon out
  carrying spare ST
2. Importance of careful washing of genital area because of odour
3. Old Wives' Tales
  can't wash your hair
  can't have a bath or shower
  can't swim or exercise
  people always know when you have one
4. Disposal of ST or tampon
	(a) Show a selection of different sorts of sanitary pads and tampons and how they are worn
	(b) Where girls can get a pad in your location; outside?
	(c) Keep a record and mark a calendar—personal responsibility

PERSONAL HYGIENE

Topic	Approaches
EMISSION HYGIENE FOR MALES	
1 Importance of cleaning penis and thighs after 'wet dream' or masturbation 2. Washing underpants/pyjama trousers as necessary	

REFERENCES: PERSONAL HYGIENE

BOOKS

Abbott, M. (undated). *Growing Up Young*. Larkfield, Kent: Kimberley-Clark Ltd.
Holt, A. and Randell, J. (1975). *Come Clean*. Cambridge: Cambridge University Press.
Schools Council Project (1977). *Get Clean*. Unit 7 of "Think Well" series. Sunbury-on-Thames: Nelson.

FILMS, SLIDES, VIDEO (for addresses of distributors see page 185)

About Your Feet	31 frame film strip and teachers' notes. Educational Audio Visual Ltd.
Educating Mentally Handicapped People	Slides or film strips. Camera Talks.
2. The Picture of Health	
3. Having a Period	
The Healthy Way in Wonderland	American film strips, cassettes and
Rub-a-dub-dub	teachers' notes. Slide Centre.
The Neat Bird	
The Wizard of Good Appearance	
Let's Go—and Get Ready	20 minute video or film of the BBC
—and Look After Our Teeth	programme. Record Off Air *or* Concord Films.

MISCELLANEOUS

Are You A Stinker?	Health Education Council Leaflet.
Self Care	ESN(S) Consortium
1. Cleaning my teeth	18 laminated colour photos and 6 pads A4 tear-off sheets
2. Coping with my period	9 laminated b/w photos
3. Washing my hands	12 laminated colour photos

164

Growing Up

The physical and emotional changes that come with puberty can bewilder and confuse youngsters, normal and mentally handicapped. Teaching and discussion should be centred on the *normality* of these changes, with practical pointers as to how teenagers can cope with these new and sometimes surprising and embarrassing consequences of developing maturity.

Topic	*Approaches*
PHYSICAL CHANGES	

1. Changes in girls
    shape
    breasts
    body hair
    periods
    sweat glands
	(a) Have plenty of pictures to show

2. Changes in boys
    shape
    voice breaks
    body hair
    erections/emissions
    penis grows
    sweat glands	

3. Possible 'problems'
    acne—so skin care
    growth spurt—may become
        clumsy
    underarm odour—so careful
        washing
    embarrassment at voice
        breaking
    irregular first few periods	

Topic	Approaches
EMOTIONAL CHANGES	

1. New ideas and interests
2. Moods
3. Day dreaming
4. Falling in love
    love/infatuation/crushes
5. Sexual feelings
    boys get erections and 'wet'
    dreams—personal hygiene
    and how to behave when an
    embarrassing erection
    happens
    girls spend a lot of time
    thinking about boys
	(a) Cut out magazine pictures
	    showing different kinds of
	    love, eg parent for child,
	    husband and wife, person for
	    object etc.
	(b) Role play different moods.

Topic	Approaches
MENSTRUATION	
1. What are periods? ⎱ boys (men) should 2. Why do women ⎰ have general information have periods? ⎰ about these topics 3. Hygiene aspects 4. Irregular periods	*Link* to: THE HUMAN BODY PERSONAL HYGIENE

Topic	Approaches
MASTURBATION	

1. What is masturbation?
    rubbing or stroking clitoris
    or penis until orgasm
2. Why do people masturbate?
    a natural function
    to feel nice
    to relax
    comforting themselves
3. Does it harm people?
    dispelling of "old wives' tales"
    stop if your skin is sore
    might get into trouble if done
    in public
4. Privacy
    designating private areas
    the law—"indecent exposure"
	(a) List places which are private
	    in the living situation of the
	    group members, and areas
	    which are public. Other staff
	    to be involved in designating
	    private areas and respecting
	    these.

REFERENCES: GROWING UP

BOOKS

Heath Education Council (no date). *How We Grow Up*. Free booklet.
Hemming, J. and Maxwell, Z. (eds.) (1975). *Achieving Sexual Maturity* and *Growing Up*. London: Macmillan.
Johnson, V. and Williams, T. (1980). *Good Health*. Book 2. Sunbury-on-Thames: Nelson.
Mayle, P. (1978). *What's Happening To Me?* London: Macmillan.
Schools Council Project (1977). *My Self* and *One of Many*. Units 1 and 2 of "Think Well" series. Sunbury-on-Thames: Nelson.

FILMS, SLIDES, VIDEO (for addresses of distributors see page 185)

Educating Mentally Handicapped People	42 Slides or film strip. Camera Talks.
3. Having a Period	
Good Health	15 minute video or 16mm film. Central TV
10. What Next?	(formerly ATV) *or* Rank Film Library.
Growing Up	15 slides, cassette and teachers' notes. No longer available from the BBC, but Education Resource Centres may have a copy.
It's Not What You Do	5 × 20 minute video cassettes. ILEA.
Unit 3: Emotions	
10. Love	
11. Hate	
12. Fear	
13. Grief	
14. Joy	
Living and Growing	15 minute videos. Grampian TV.
2. The Same but Different	
3. Physiology of Sex	
Sexuality and the Mentally Handicapped	Set of Winifred Kempton's teaching slides. Available for hire from FPA *or* SPOD:
II. Male Puberty	Purchase from Concord films *or*
III. Female Puberty	E. Patterson Assoc. Ltd.

MISCELLANEOUS

Living Well	Work cards and teachers' notes.
And How Are We Feeling Today?	Health Education Council.
Support Group	
The Many Faces of Youth	12 photoposters (12 ins. × 18 ins.) and teachers' notes. Taskmaster.
See How You Feel	20 discussion and 30 domino cards. Learning Development Aids.

167

Adulthood

Being an adult (over 18 in law) usually involves taking responsibility for all areas of life—where we work, live, who we live with, friends, personal appearance, etc. By definition, people who are mentally handicapped may never attain responsibility for all these areas; but incompetence in one area does *not* necessarily mean an overall inability to make sensible decisions about things which affect their lives. In a residential setting it is very easy for staff to assume for the residents many of the responsibilities of adulthood.

Again, this module prompts a look at the areas where people over 18 could be helped to assume more personal responsibilities. This is particularly important in the matter of sexual behaviour—we cannot, and of course should not, oversee every move that the mentally handicapped people in our care make, but we *should* make sure that no one is ignorant of the fact that unprotected sexual intercourse can result in a pregnancy, that promiscuous behaviour can mean V.D., that no one should approach a child sexually or another adult without their consent.

Topic	*Approaches*
MEN AND WOMEN	

1. Physical differences between men and women
    body shape
    breasts
    reproductive system
    hair growth
	Link to: GROWING UP module
	(a) Pictures from magazines of different sexes, ages, races, appearances.
	(b) Divide into pairs, name 2 things the same about you both, 2 things that are different.

2. Similarities:
    heart
    brain
    eyes
    legs, etc.	

3. Differences and similarities between people of the same sex:
    mental and physical abilities
    physical appearance
    all share certain characteristics (including needing love and affection)
    yet each person is unique	

4. Differences and similarities between people of other races:
    colour
    hair
    facial characteristics
    customs
    religion	

5. What would happen if we all looked alike?	

Topic	Approaches
ADULT RESPONSIBILITIES	

1. Personal
   health
   hygiene
   appropriate dress
   care of possessions
   choice of friends
   citizenship, eg voting, concept
   of government
2. Financial
   Personal Income
   wages for work done
   State benefits and allowances
   Expenditure
   day-to-day necessities
   luxuries
   income tax
   Saving
   for special spending, eg
   holiday, record player
   for a rainy day
3. Sexual
   Every time a mature boy and
   girl (ie boy who has erections
   with emission, and girl who
   menstruates) have intercourse, there is a chance they
   will start a baby, therefore
   contraception
   Why do people make love?
   casual; "in love", commitment; pleasure; to make a
   baby; comfort; excitement;
   careless
   Dangers of V.D.—responsibility to self and partner.
   The Law
   (i) A boy or man who sexually
   takes by force an unwilling
   partner may be charged
   with *rape*.

(a) What responsibilities has
growth brought the group?
Is there an area in which they
could be helped and encouraged
to assume personal control.

(b) Keep records for a week of
personal income and expenditure (staff to help record as
necessary).

(c) Family Planning—demonstration kit of contraceptive
devices.

(d) Correct misconceptions about
'safe' ways and times to have
sexual intercourse, eg standing
up; just before a woman's
period.

(e) Collect examples of advertisements which use sex to
sell products.

(f) Visit local V.D. clinic for talk
by nurse or doctor.

(g) Role play moral choices, eg
you see someone stealing in
a shop, what do you do? Your
friend dares you to do something you know is wrong and
calls you a sissy/coward when
you at first refuse. What
happens next?

(h) Filling in different forms.

Topic	Approaches
ADULT RESPONSIBILITIES *cont.*	

ADULT RESPONSIBILITIES
cont.
- (ii) Handling, fondling, kissing unwilling partner may be *indecent assault*.
- (iii) No adult may play sexually with, or attempt intercourse with a child (under 16)
- (iv) All sexual behaviour involving the genitals must be in private
- (v) Law on homosexuality— privacy; no partner under 21 or severely mentally handicapped.
4. Legal
      contracts—hire purchase, TV rental, etc.
      making a will
      legal aid
5. Moral choices
      what makes some things right to do, some wrong?
            the law
            does it hurt other people?
      do you sometimes do wrong things, even when you know it's wrong?
      what makes us do this?
6. Self-control and outside authority

Topic	Approaches
ADULT RELATIONSHIPS	
1. Reminder of girl/boy friends from GROWING UP	(a) Get the group to put in priority order the qualities they might look for in a partner. Show differences.
2. Marriage: what keeps partners together? what may split them up?	(b) Marriage patterns in other countries.
3. What does marriage mean? legally in personal terms—needs of self and partner advantages/disadvantages	(c) Compile a "problem page" from magazine readers' letters. What advice would the group give in each case?
4. Does marriage always mean parenthood? family planning	(d) Getting a mother to bring in a young baby, and a toddler to the group, discussing aspects of child care.
5. Parenthood physical and emotional needs of young children over the years	(e) Use a cassette orecording of a young baby crying, and talk with it on for 10 minutes, then switch it off—you can't turn a baby off!
6. Homosexuality legal position in the eyes of society a personal choice	

Topic	Approaches
GROWING OLD	
1. What happens to our bodies as we grow older? appearance sight/hearing energy/speed more easily damaged	(a) Pictures of old people
2. What happens to our minds when we grow older? more forgetful harder to concentrate	
3. How can we compensate?	
4. Menopause how the female body changes physical symptoms emotional feelings medication	

REFERENCES: ADULTHOOD

BOOKS

Althea (1975). *A Baby in the Family*. Cambridge: Dinosaur Publications.

Andry, A.C. and Schepp, S. (1969). *How Babies Are Made*. London: Time-Life International.

Anglund, J.W. (1960). *Love is a Special Way of Feeling*. London: Collins.

Baldwin, D. (1978). *Then and Now*. London: Longman Child Development Series.

Baldwin, D. (1979). *Understanding Your Baby*. Revised edition. London: Ebury Press.

Brook Advisory Centres Unit (undated). *A Look at Safe Sex*.

Chovil, C. and Jones, E.G. (1977). *How Did I Grow?* London: BBC Publications.

Fagerstrom, G. and Hansson, G. (1979). *Our New Baby*. London: Macdonald Educational.

Fox, D. and Smith, J. (1977). *Facts for Life: Family Matters*. London: Macdonald Educational.

Hemming, J. and Maxwell, Z. (eds.) (1975). *A Baby Arrives, Growing Up,* and *Achieving Sexual Maturity*. London: Macmillan.

Holt, A. and Randall, J. (1976). *The Two of Us*. Cambridge: Cambridge University Press.

Mayle, P. (1978). *Where Did I Come From?* London: Macmillan.

Mayle, P. (1978). *Will I Like It?* London: W.H. Allen.

Schools Council Project (1977). *Knowing About Others*. Unit 7 of "All About Me" series. *One of Many*. Unit 2 of "Think Well" series. Sunbury-on-Thames: Nelson.

Sheffield, M. (1973). *Where Do Babies Come From?* London: Jonathan Cape. (Education Resource Centres may have a copy of the BBC radiovision filmstrip based on the book. It is now no longer available for purchase.)

Spiers, H. (1971). *How You Began*. London: J.M. Dent & Sons.

Swindells, A.P. (1977). *Sex*. St. Albans: Hart Davis Educational.

Ward, B. (1976). *Sex and Life*. London: Macdonald Educational.

FILMS, SLIDES, VIDEO (for addresses of distributors see p. 185)

Are We Still Going To The Movies?	16 mm 14-minute American colour film. McGraw Hill Book (UK) Ltd. *or* Concord Films.
Birth	24 slides or film strip. Camera Talks.
The Child's World	20-minute videos. ILEA.
1. Birthright	
2. Changing Needs	
3. Communication	
4. Safety	
5. The World Outside	
Educating Mentally Handicapped People	Camera Talks.
1. Behave Yourself!	50 slides or film strip.

Facts for Life
1. Expecting a Baby
2. Jenny is Born
3. More about Childbirth
4. The Start of Life
5. A Baby in the House
6. Early Years
7. Take Care!
8. Special Needs
   The Least You Can Do

20-minutes videos or 16 mm films.
Available from Granada TV *or*
Concord Films.

Good Health
1. Everybody is Different

15-minute video or 16mm film. Central TV
(formerly ATV) *or* Rank Film Library.

How Babies Are Born

16mm 10-minute British colour film.
Eothen Films International Ltd.

Human Growth

16mm 20-minute American colour film.
Concord Films.

Living and Growing
1. Family and Friends
4. Loving and Caring
5. Prenatal Care
6. Preparing for Birth
7. Postnatal Care
8. It's Your Life

15-minute videos. Grampian TV.

Making Love

16mm 25-minute British colour film.
Guild Sound and Vision Ltd.

Menopause

30 slides or film strip with cassette and
teachers' notes. Camera Talks.

Merry-go-Round
1. Beginning
2. Birth
3. Full Circle

BBC Enterprises *or* Videorecord
off air.

Sexuality and the Mentally Handicapped
IV. Social Behavior
V. Human Reproduction
VII. Venereal Disease and Sexual
     Health
VIII. Marriage
IX. Parenting

Sets of Winifred Kempton's teaching
slides. Available for hire from FPA *or*
SPOD. Purchase from Concord Films *or*
E. Patterson Assoc. Ltd.

You Can't Have One Without The Other

16mm 25-minute British B/W film about
birth control. Concord Films.

MISCELLANEOUS

Contraceptive Display Kit

Sample of contraceptives from the Family
Planning Association.

It'll Never be the Same

Longman Think Strip on parenthood.
Purchase in sets of 10 with teacher's
notes.

Marriage for Life?

Large chart (76 × 100 cm) and teacher's
notes. Pictorial Charts.

174

| *Talking Points* | Set 2: Life. Set of 25 B/W photocards (10 ins. × 8 ins.). Photographic Teaching Materials. |
| *Your Child* | Large Chart (76 × 100 cm) with teacher's notes. Pictorial Charts. |

Interpersonal Relationships

Interpersonal relationships involve complex social skills, and as we know from everyday experiences, some people are better at establishing and maintaining cordial contacts than others. Intelligence is not necessarily an important factor, many a clever person goes through life putting people's backs up, ignoring everyone's feelings but his own.

Teachers will be aware of the personal history of the individuals in the group. There will be those with poor family backgrounds and relationships which are destructive. Where the mentally handicapped individuals are over eighteen emphasis should be that adults are usually independent of their parents, while remaining on friendly terms.

The focus of the module is simple—the way we behave towards others has an effect on the way they treat us. The more considerate, thoughtful and tolerant we are, the nicer we are to be with and the more people enjoy our company. If we are selfish, rude and badly behaved, friends are few and life is not so enjoyable.

Topic	*Approaches*
GOOD AND BAD MANNERS	
1. Why bother with good manners? makes life easier and more pleasant	(a) Ask for examples of good and bad manners; of selfishness and selflessness.
2. Social skills introductions and shaking hands saying goodbye taking 'turns' in conversation invitations—issuing, accepting, refusing saying "no" politely queueing—bus stops, shops, etc.	(b) Role play: good and bad manners.
3. Table manners	
4. Politeness to older people	

Topic	*Approaches*
OTHER PEOPLE'S FEELINGS	
1. Recognising how other people are feeling by their expressions	(a) Use pictures from magazines etc. showing different emotions by facial expression and body posture.
2. What does it mean to be tolerant? of another's handicaps of another's feelings	(b) Miming different emotions, group to guess.
3. What does it mean to be selfish/to be unselfish	(c) Role play: brief 4 people separately, one to insist on watching football match on TV, one to have headache and want a quiet evening, one wanting to hear new record, one wanting to play a card game needing 4 people.
4. What does it mean to "use" someone? eg very friendly with someone when you want to borrow something, ignore them otherwise	

176

Topic	*Approaches*
RELATIONSHIPS WITH OTHERS	
1. With our family 　what do we expect from them? 　how realistic are our expecta- 　tions? 　how do we behave towards 　them? 　what do families quarrel about?	(a) Role play family situations 　eg Mum coming home from 　shopping or work expecting 　tea ready, son or daughter 　just listening to records.
2. With staff in the school/hospital/ 　hostel 　what do students/residents 　expect from them? 　what do they expect from 　students/residents? 　how do you behave? 　what upsets staff/students/ 　residents? 　making rules—are they fair?	(b) Make a set of rules for your 　home/class/hostel/ward. How 　do these differ from existing 　rules? (c) Make a list of qualities we 　look for in a friend. Put your 　list in order of priority. (d) How good a friend are you? 　What do you have to offer?
3. With our friends 　why do we have friends? 　what do we expect from 　friends? 　loyalty 　how do we behave? 　do friends quarrel?	(e) Trust games: 　(i) leading someone blindfold 　around furniture and obstacles 　that have been rearranged. 　(ii) make a very tight standing 　circle, one person in centre 　with eyes closed and hands by 　sides. People in circle gently 　move person in centre back- 　wards and forwards and from
4. With an employer 　what do we expect from an 　employer? 　how do we behave?	side to side, always catching 　him and gently moving him on. 　Special care is needed to take 　account of physical handicaps 　of participants.
5. Your effect on other people 　does how you behave make any 　difference?	(e) Role play work situations—eg 　arriving late and apologising; 　asking for time off. (g) Role play: asking someone to 　do something for you politely, 　asking rudely.

Topic	Approaches
GIRL FRIENDS/BOY FRIENDS	
1. What do we look for in a girl/boy friend?	(a) List the qualities you would look for in a girl/boy friend. Is being pretty/handsome as important as being kind?
2. How do we behave?	
3. Going out on a date	
4. Going steady—what does this mean?	(b) Role play behaviour with girl/boy friend. Behaviour in public and in private.
5. What is love? different meanings of the word	(c) Role play going out on a date—asking/accepting, getting ready, checking money, home telephone number, behaviour on date, saying goodnight.
	(d) List different meanings of "love".

Topic	Approaches
COMMUNICATION	
1. How do we let other people know how we feel?	(a) Role play and mime, showing anger, happiness, sadness, jealousy, puzzlement, etc.
(a) by speech/sign language	
(b) by action	(b) In a circle pass round a frown, a smile, a funny face, etc.
(c) by facial expression	
(d) by body movement	(c) In a circle pass round an imaginary hot plate, a sleeping baby, a baby who has just been sick down you, a letter with good news, etc.
2. The importance of listening, and paying attention, to others	
3. Misunderstandings how do these happen? how can we correct them?	(d) In pairs, one the actor, the other the mirror. The mirror has to copy exactly the movements of the actor.
	(e) In a circle one person starts a story, points to another who has to continue, and so on.

INTERPERSONAL RELATIONSHIPS

Topic	Approaches
EMOTIONS	
1. What are emotions and how do they affect behaviour?	(a) Get students to finish sentences:
2. Being moody	If I am angry I ....
how do we feel?	If I am happy I ....
how do others treat us?	If I am sad I ....
3. When something has upset you, how do you behave?	If I am lonely I ....
4. When you are angry, what do you do?	(b) Role play: someone sulking, others trying to join in an activity; being angry and losing temper; being angry and controlling temper.
5. How do people control their tempers?	(c) What makes each group member happy/sad/angry etc?

REFERENCES: INTERPERSONAL RELATIONSHIPS

BOOKS

Anglund, J.W. (1960). *Love is a Special Way of Feeling*. London: Collins.

Holt, A. and Brand, J. (1976). *The Two of Us*. Cambridge: Cambridge University Press.

Jennings, S. (1973). *Remedial Drama*. Pitman.

Johnson, V. and Williams, T. (1980). *Good Health*. Book 2. Sunbury-on-Thames: Nelson.

Mayle, P. (1978). *Will I Like It?* London: W.H. Allen.

McPhail, P., Middleton, D. and Ingram, D. (1978). *Startline*. Schools Council Moral Education 8–13 Project. London: Longman.

Roberts, R. (1978). *Families*. One of 8 booklets matching programmes in the ATV Series "Alive and Kicking". Sunbury-on-Thames: Nelson.

Schools Council Project (1977). *Knowing About Others*. Unit 7 of "All About Me" series. Sunbury-on-Thames: Nelson.

Warren, B. (1981). *Drama Games for Mentally Handicapped People*. London: National Society for Mentally Handicapped Children and Adults.

FILMS, SLIDES, VIDEO (for addresses of distributors see p. 185)

Are We Still Going to the Movies?	16 mm 14-minute American colour film. McGraw Hill Books (UK) Ltd. *or* Concord Films.
Educating Mentally Handicapped People	50 slides or film strip, cassette and teachers' notes. Camera Talks.
1. Behave Yourself!	
Good Health	15-minute video or 16mm film. Central TV (formerly ATV) *or* Rank Film Library.
12. Summer Camp (film entitled "Three of Us")	

Good Manners Are Me	Film strips and cassettes. View Tech
Me, Myself and I	Audiovisual Media.
I Live With People	
I Have Friends	
Living and Growing	15-minute videos. Grampian TV.
1. Family and Friends	
4. Loving and Caring	
Me and My Family	Set of 6 film strips with cassettes and
It's not Fair!	teachers' notes. View Tech
Why Can't I?	Audiovisual Media.
Please Listen!	
Angry Words, Angry Feelings	
It's Your Fault!	
That's Mine!	
My Feelings Count!	Four American film strips and teachers'
I Wonder	notes. Fergus Davidson Ltd.
The Me I Like	
When Things Go Wrong	
When I Feel Afraid	
Sexuality and the Mentally Handicapped	Sets of Winifred Kempton's teaching
IV. Social Behavior	slides. Available for hire from FPA *or*
	SPOD. Purchase from Concord Films
	or E. Patterson Assoc. Ltd.
Values: Right or Wrong	Six American film strips, cassettes and
Why Rules?	teachers' notes. Fergus Davidson Ltd.
What is Responsibility?	
What is Honesty?	
Why Play Fair?	
What is Yours, What is Mine?	
What is Appreciating Others?	

MISCELLANEOUS

Multi-Ethnic People Puzzles	Two sets of 8 puzzles (22×28 cm.), 1 on
	faces and 1 on the whole body.
	Taskmaster.
People Puzzles	Two sets of 8 puzzles, black or white
	family group. Taskmaster.
This is Me	Thirty-two coloured cards (28×23 cm.)
	with a picture on each side. Taskmaster.

Self-concept

Mentally handicapped people often have a very poor self-concept and low self-esteem. They are nearly always on the *receiving* end of care and never allowed to play an important part in decisions affecting their lives. Their capacity for independent thought and decision-making is not encouraged and the helplessness and acquiescent behaviour which result reinforces the parents and professionals that here is someone who will always be as dependent as a child. When 'goodness' becomes equated with 'do as you are told' it is not surprising that retarded individuals lack the personal initiative which stems from self-confidence.

This module aims at helping students to achieve a more realistic image of themselves, and to encourage them to be more assertative in their dealings with the people around them.

Topic	*Approaches*
GENDER IDENTIFICATION	
1. Reminder of the physical differences between men and women	(a) Magazine pictures
2. Are there differences in behaviour between men and women?	(b) list what hobbies men/women like to do: very many are shared

3. Traditional roles
  male—breadwinner, provider
  female—child care
	(c) List the characteristics traditionally linked to men eg "strong", "don't show emotion", "the boss". List the

4. Contemporary roles
  sharing tasks
  equal pay, equal rights
	characteristics traditionally linked to women eg "emotional", "weak", "looks after the home". Do these still apply?

Topic	Approaches
PORTRAIT OF MYSELF	

1. Measurment and observation
    height
    weight
    colour of hair/eyes
    etc.
2. Self-portrait—drawing
3. My family
    family tree, perhaps with
      photos
	(a) Each individual completes a
	    simple chart:
	    my Christian/first name is:
	    my surname/last name is:
	    age:
	    sex:
	    height:
	    weight:
	    colour of hair:
	    colour of eyes:
	    clothing size:
	    shoe size:
	    Who is the tallest/shortest/
	    oldest, etc?
	(b) Draws outline round each
	    individual on large sheet of
	    paper to show different sizes
	    and shapes.
	(c) Making family trees, perhaps
	    with photos.

Topic	*Approaches*
PERSONAL POTENTIAL AND LIMITATIONS	

1. Things I can do well
2. Things I find difficult
3. My good qualities
4. My bad qualities
5. My handicaps
6. Can I make life better for myself?
	(a) Make lists under each heading.
	    Do other members of the
	    group agree or disagree?

Topic	*Approaches*
SELF ESTEEM	

<table>
<tr>
<td>

1. What sort of person am I?
2. Standing up for myself
    in public places eg shop,
      restaurant
    door-to-door salesmen
    sexual exploitation
      sexual advance by a stranger
      sexual advance by someone
        known but not liked

</td>
<td>

(a) Recap of personal potential and limitations.
(b) Tape record different voice tones, eg hesitant, assured, angry, excited.
(c) Videotape sessions—allow people to see and judge their own appearance, behaviour and effect on others.
(d) (i) Role play: a café advertises "today's special" for a set price. Four people have it. When the waiter/waitress brings the bill an extra item has been charged. Payment is demanded—do the four notice the extra? Pay? Complain? Ask to see the manager?
(ii) In a crowded supermarket there is only one check-out operating. You only have a few items in your basket; the woman behind has a trolleyful. She asks you "Do you mind if I go before you. I have a bus to catch in five minutes". You have a friend outside who has already been waiting a long time for you. Do you let the woman go in front of you or refuse?
(iii) A door-to-door salesman calls when you are alone at home. He is selling radios and cassette players. You have been saving for a radio but haven't enough money. He asks you to sign a form for credit terms.
(iv) A man you don't know offers you a lift to your home. What do you say?

</td>
</tr>
</table>

REFERENCES: SELF CONCEPT

BOOKS

Jennings, S. (1973). *Remedial Drama*. Pitman.
Johnson, V. and Williams, T. (1979). *Good Health*. Book 1. Sunbury-on-Thames: Nelson.
McPhail, P., Middleton, D. and Ingram, D.(1978). *Startline*. Schools Council Moral Education 8–13 Project. London: Longman.
Schools Council Project (1977). *Finding Out About Myself*. Unit 1 of "All About Me" series. *Myself*. Unit 1 of "Think Well" series. Sunbury-on-Thames: Nelson.
Seuss, Dr. and McKie, R. (1973). *My Book All About Me*. London: Collins.

FILMS (for addresses of distributors see p. 185)

How Do You Feel?	14 frame film strip. Fergus Davidson Ltd.
Living and Growing 2. The Same but Different	15-minute video. Grampian TV.
My Feelings Count! I Wonder The Me I Like When Things Go Wrong I Feel Afraid	American film strips with teachers' notes.. Fergus Davidson Ltd.
Myself and Me What Do I Look Like? How Do I Feel? What Do I Like To Do? What Do I Dream About?	American film strips and cassettes. Fergus Davidson Ltd.

MISCELLANEOUS

Body Imagery	Mark on/wipe off cards. Living and Learning.
The Many Faces of Youth	12 photoposters (12 ins. × 18 ins.) and teachers' notes. Taskmaster.
People Puzzles	Two sets of eight puzzles. Black or white family groups. Taskmaster.
See How You Feel	Twenty discussion and domino cards. Learning Development Aids.
This is Me	Thirty-two coloured cards (28 × 23 cm) with a picture on each side. Taskmaster.

Elwyn Institutes (1975). *Personal Adjustment Training*. Vol. I, Basic Course; Vol. II, Assertive Training; Vol. III, Appropriate Behavior Training. Elwyn, Pennsylvania.

DISTRIBUTORS

BBC Enterprises, Villiers House, Broadway, Ealing, London.

BBC Publications, School Order Section, 144–152 Bermondsey Stret, London SE1 3TH.

British Institute of Mental Handicap, Wolverhampton Road, Kidderminster, Worcestershire DY10 3PP.

Brook Advisory Centres Unit, 10 Albert Street, Birmingham B4 7UD.

Camera Talks Ltd., 31 North Row, London W1R 2EN.

Central Independent Television, Broad Street, Birmingham B1 2JP.

Concord Films Council Ltd., 201 Felixstowe Road, Ipswich IP3 9BJ.

Educational Audio Visual Ltd., Butterley Street, Leeds LS10 1AX.

Eothen Films Ltd., EMI Film Studios, Shenley Road, Boreham Wood, Herts WD6 1JG.

ESN(S) Consortium (ILEA), Jack Tizard School, Finlay Street, London SW6 6HB.

Family Planning Association, 27-35 Mortimer Street, London W.1.

Fergus Davidson Associates Ltd., 1 Bensham Lane, Croydon CR0 2RU.

Grampian Television Ltd., Queen's Cross, Aberdeen, AB9 2XJ.

Granada Television Ltd., Manchester M60 9EA.

Guild Sound and Vision Ltd., 85-129 Oundle Road, Peterborough PE2 9PZ.

HMSO , PO Box 569, London SE1 9NH.

ILEA Learning Materials Service, Highbury, Station Road, London N1 1SB.

Kimberley-Clark Ltd., Larkfield, Kent.

Learning Development Aids, Aware House, Duke Street, Wisbech, Cambs PE13 2AE.

Living and Learning, as LDA above.

Longman Group Ltd., Burnt Mill, Harlow, Essex CM20 1BR.

McGraw Hill Books (UK) Ltd., Shoppenhangers Road, Maidenhead, Berks SL6 2QL.

Edward Patterson Associates Ltd., 68 Copers Cope Road, Beckenham, Kent.

Photographic Teaching Materials, 23 Horn Street, Winslow, Buckingham MK18 3AP.

Pictorial Charts Educational Trust, 27 Kirchen Road, London W13 0UD.

Rank Film Library, PO Box 70, Great West Road, Brentford, Middlesex TW8 9HR.

The Slide Centre, 143 Chatham Road, London SW11 6SR.

SPOD, The Diorama, 14 Peto Place, London NW1 4DT.

Taskmaster, Morris Road, Clarendon Park, Leicester LE2 6BR.

View Tech Audiovisual Media, 122 Goldcrest Road, Chipping Sodbury, Bristol BS7C 6XN

CHAPTER 9

Teaching Programmes and Training Techniques

Ann Craft

Teaching Programmes

Education of the mentally handicapped members of our society has undergone, and is undergoing, many changes. We now no longer believe that any child is 'ineducable', teachers and psychologists have sought for new methods, approaches, strategies to educate those whose disabilities inhibit normal learning. Whelan and Speake (1979) in their book *Learning to Cope* outline ways in which mentally handicapped adolescents and adults can be helped to learn social skills and appropriate behaviour. Their work is very relevant to the theme of this book, and the first section of this chapter draws heavily on their material.

Assessment

Before embarking on a teaching programme, we need to know the strengths and the gaps in repertoires of behaviour. Whelan and Speake's Scale for Assessing Coping Skills* covers a very wide range of behaviours. Here we reproduce that part of the scale relating to interpersonal skills (pp 188–91).

From the scale it is possible to easily see what the present position is and what needs to be done. If columns (1) and (5) are ticked for a particular skill, then the mentally handicapped person can, and does, function adequately. Parents and care staff may need to discuss what constitutes 'adequately', and a check is suggested (p. 187). If the numbers in the boxes are not the same then there is a target to work towards.

If column (1) is ticked with column (6) then although the skill is present, it is under-used. Items ticked under columns (2) and (3)

---

* Full scale available from Copewell Publications, 29 Worcester Road, Alkrington, Middleton, Manchester M24 1PA.

Frequency	This is how often it happens	This is how often we would like it to happen
(1) Never		
(2) Few times a year		
(3) Once a month		
(4) Few times a month		
(5) Once a week		
(6) Few times a week		
(7) Once a day		
(8) More than once a day		

mean that training is needed to develop or foster a skill. A tick in column (4) means assessment is necessary. A tick in column (7) might lead us to re-examine the environment and opportunities open to the mentally handicapped individual.

Goal Setting

Targets must be discussed with the mentally handicapped person, as there has to be something he or she *wants* to learn or accept responsibility for. Goals should be precise items of behaviour, we may defeat ourselves at the outset if we set vague and all-embracing targets such as 'become more responsible' or 'improvement in personal hygiene'. Many discrete behaviours are involved, and it is these that must be isolated as goals. For example, an adolescent boy might need to learn how to tell the time before he can accept responsibility for getting home at a set hour or keeping an appointment punctually. A girl may need specific lessons in washing, rinsing, setting and drying her hair, which is only one part of personal hygiene, but one step towards the whole.

Rewards

A reward tells the learner what he has just done was correct, it also makes it more likely that the action will be repeated on other occasions. Whenever possible, the reward should directly follow the correct behaviour, so that they are associated in the mind of the learner. Verbal praise can be a powerful reward, especially coupled with a sense of personal satisfaction and pleasure that comes when the mentally handicapped person has chosen the goal for him or herself. The rewards will obviously differ between individuals and between age groups. A child might be rewarded by a sweet or a hand-clap, but it is more adult for silence itself to be the reward,

ITEM	1 Can do without help or supervision	2 Can do but only with help or supervision	3 Cannot yet do	4 Do not yet know whether he can do	5 Uses this ability an adequate amount	6 Does not use this an adequate amount	7 There is no opportunity to do this
INTERPERSONAL							
Personal knowledge							
(a) Knows full name, address, sex	☐	☐	☐	☐	☐	☐	☐
(b) Knows age and birthday and telephone number (where appropriate)	☐	☐	☐	☐	☐	☐	☐
(c) Knows nationality, name of country and religion	☐ ☐	☐ ☐	☐ ☐	☐ ☐	☐ ☐	☐ ☐	☐ ☐
(d) Can name and describe members of immediate family							
(e) Has fairly realistic idea of own strengths and limitiations	☐	☐	☐	☐	☐	☐	☐
Conversation							
(a) Uses basic social conversation, 'Hello', 'good morning', 'how are you' etc.	☐	☐	☐	☐	☐	☐	☐
(b) Relates experiences, recent events, etc.	☐	☐	☐	☐	☐	☐	☐
(c) Talks about subject of interest to person concerned	☐ ☐	☐ ☐	☐ ☐	☐ ☐	☐ ☐	☐ ☐	☐ ☐
(d) Seeks other person's advice or opinion							
(e) Knows when someone is getting bored and brings conversation to an end, or changes topic	☐	☐	☐	☐	☐	☐	☐

ITEM	1 Can do without help or supervision	2 Can do but only with help or supervision	3 Cannot yet do	4 Do not yet know whether he can do	5 Uses this ability an adequate amount	6 Does not use this an adequate amount	7 There is no opportunity to do this
Social graces							
(a) Says 'please' and 'thank you'	☐	☐	☐	☐	☐	☐	☐
(b) Greets others in appropriate way	☐	☐	☐	☐	☐	☐	☐
(c) Takes turn, waits patiently	☐	☐	☐	☐	☐	☐	☐
(d) Knocks on doors before entering, or excuses self, where appropriate	☐	☐	☐	☐	☐	☐	☐
(e) Can take hint when someone wants to leave or wants privacy	☐	☐	☐	☐	☐	☐	☐
Friendships							
(a) Generally tries to get along with others	☐	☐	☐	☐	☐	☐	☐
(b) Shares or lends possessions with discretion	☐	☐	☐	☐	☐	☐	☐
(c) Shows warmth or affection, kindness and sympathy	☐	☐	☐	☐	☐	☐	☐
(d) Keeps in touch with friend, remembers birthday, etc.	☐	☐	☐	☐	☐	☐	☐
(e) Considers friends' feelings, offers help where possible	☐	☐	☐	☐	☐	☐	☐

189

ITEM	1 Can do without help or super-vision	2 Can do but only with help or supervision	3 Cannot yet do	4 Do not yet know whether he can do	5 Use this ability an adequate amount	6 Does not uses this an adequate amount	7 There is no opportunity to do this
Leisure—group activities							
(a) Enjoys being in the company of others, going to party, dance or disco	☐	☐	☐	☐	☐	☐	☐
(b) Attends club or social centre	☐	☐	☐	☐	☐	☐	☐
(c) Goes to cinema, theatre, sporting or athletic event	☐	☐	☐	☐	☐	☐	☐
(d) Takes part in team games	☐	☐	☐	☐	☐	☐	☐
(e) Takes part in drama, concert, amateur theatrical, band or choir	☐	☐	☐	☐	☐	☐	☐
Telephone							
(a) Answers phone and calls appropriate person or takes simple message	☐	☐	☐	☐	☐	☐	☐
(b) Answers phone and carries on simple conversation	☐	☐	☐	☐	☐	☐	☐
(c) Dials and obtains a required number (written down) and asks for person concerned, including emergency	☐	☐	☐	☐	☐	☐	☐
(d) Uses a call-box for well-known numbers	☐	☐	☐	☐	☐	☐	☐
(e) Uses a telephone directory with some success	☐	☐	☐	☐	☐	☐	☐

ITEM	1 Can do without help or supervision	2 Can do but only with help or supervision	3 Cannot yet do	4 Do not yet know whether he can do	5 Uses this ability an adequate amount	6 Does not use this an adequate amount	7 There is no opportunity to do this
Responsibility							
(a) Aware of rules and the need to keep them (safety, honesty, punctuality, hygiene, etc.)	☐	☐	☐	☐	☐	☐	☐
Accepts criticism where appropriate	☐	☐	☐	☐	☐	☐	☐
(b) Anticipates the consequence of own actions	☐	☐	☐	☐	☐	☐	☐
(c) Accepts blame for own mistakes	☐	☐	☐	☐	☐	☐	☐
(d) Shows concern for the safety or welfare of others	☐	☐	☐	☐	☐	☐	☐
Sexual knowledge and behaviour							
(a) Aware of differences between men and women	☐	☐	☐	☐	☐	☐	☐
(b) Understands own sexual development, pubic hair, breasts, etc.	☐	☐	☐	☐	☐	☐	☐
(c) Knows how babies are conceived and born, in context of love and marriage	☐	☐	☐	☐	☐	☐	☐
(d) Aware of birth control, dangers of venereal disease, etc.	☐	☐	☐	☐	☐	☐	☐
(e) Behaves with responsibility and respect in relations with opposite sex (not over affectionate, or promiscuous)	☐	☐	☐	☐	☐	☐	☐

accompanied by close attention. On successful completion, a smile and praise is the reward, and in the long term what reinforces is the handing over of the responsibility for that task to the mentally handicapped individual.

Corrective remarks should be kept to a minimum, as they may discourage the learner from persevering with the task. A shake of the head or 'no' may be needed, but it is much more pleasant to be praised for what is correct, than criticised for what is wrong. The tasks should be broken down in sufficiently easy and clear stages to minimise the possible number of mistakes.

Teaching Principles

Whelan and Speake (1979) list ten principles:

(1) Insist that each operation be carried out correctly before proceeding to the next—remember that incorrect performance only results in habits which have to be unlearned.

(2) Ensure success by presenting only a small step at a time.

(3) Use simple language and clear gestures. Speak slowly and distinctly, and be consistent in your use of words.

(4) Inform the learner whether his performance is correct or not. During the early stages of learning, correct behaviour should be rewarded immediately, by saying 'Good', or 'That's right'. As the learner progresses with the task, reward him by your silence and interest, only saying 'Well done' when the task is completed.

(5) Space your teaching sessions out over time. Three sessions of 20 minutes each are likely to be more effective than one session of an hour.

(6) Once the task has been mastered, ensure that it is practised several times more. It has been found that this 'over-learning' is a powerful way of ensuring that the task will not readily be forgotten.

(7) Make full use of the different senses when teaching. Ensure that the learner not only sees, but also hears what is involved. Help him to feel the correct movements, for example, by standing behind him and 'moulding' his actions until he gets the feeling of the correct movements involved.

(8) Provide opportunities for this new knowledge or skill to be transferred to a different setting. For example, if teaching your son or daughter to make a pot of tea, perhaps he or she could

practise this in the home of a relative, using a different teapot, type of cooker, and so on.

(9) In addition to motivating the individual by pointing out the challenge which has been overcome, discuss the advantages it has for greater independence. Show your enthusiasm and admiration for the progress made, emphasising the success which this represents.

(10) Give the learner the opportunity to show others how it is done—a younger brother or sister, for example. The chance to act as a teacher is one which is greatly appreciated by many mentally handicapped people. Recent research has shown that they can be most effective teachers, and experiments in 'pyramid teaching' have proved very popular.

How do these principles apply in practice? Whelan and Speake go on to make specific suggestions for the items on the assessment chart. For example, there is an item under *Friendships*—'shares or lends possessions with discretion', and here they suggest a discussion about the difference between lending possessions and giving them to others. Also the difference between things that may be lent, like a record, and personal things like a toothbrush, which should be kept to oneself. Role play situations will help the mentally handicapped person respond appropriately when asked if something may be borrowed.

Check-lists of knowledge

It is helpful, as we have seen, to get some idea of what mentally handicapped people know and can do already, before beginning any teaching. We make our task easier by being able to build on existing knowledge and strengths. A completed check-list also gives a baseline against which we can measure progress. There are several tools available for the purpose (Fischer *et al*, 1974; Davies, 1980; Wish *et al* 1980). However, any checklist should be approached with caution. Does it make clear *who* is to do *what*, under what *conditions,* and to what *degree of success*? The danger is that checklists attempt to cover such a wide area that they use items that can be interpreted ambiguously. Terms like *identify* and *recognise* allow different raters too much latitude in assessing a subject's performance. It may be necessary to make the checklist you choose to use more precise for your purpose, so that each person that rates is quite clear what particular behaviour constitutes a correct, a partially correct, or an incorrect response. The whole purpose is defeated if one rater scores only the right name being spoken and attached to an object as correct, while another counts silently pointing to a given object as a successful completion of the task. Re-testing at a later date with different raters will only then measure the difference between the testers, and mask the progress or slipping back of the subject. Here we reproduce an outline devised by teachers of severely mentally handicapped adolescents called a *Health Education Checklist* (Cabon and Scott, ILEA 1980). Users would need to modify its items to suit their circumstances, and as indicated above, decide precisely *who* is to do *what*, under *what conditions* to what *degree of success.*

HEALTH EDUCATION CHECKLIST*

PART ONE   KNOWLEDGE OF SELF

1.1 *Parts of the body*

Can the children——?
(1) Identify common parts of the body?
(2) Identify common sex differentiating parts of the body?
(3) Distinguish between bones and skin?
(4) Recognise a skeleton?
(5) Understand how joints can move, e.g., running, jumping, bending, stretching, sitting, swimming (by using marionettes)?
(6) Experiment with movements of feet, hands, legs, arms, head, etc., to understand concept of movement?
(7) Appreciate that all parts of the body need regular exercise to keep healthy?
(8) Use their hands for a variety of tasks (strength, manipulation, deftness, sensation, etc.)?
(9) Explore the use of different senses: e.g.
smell a range of (invisible) scents
touch a number of different textures
listen to common sounds on tape
find out what it feels like to be blindfold?

1.2 *Growing*

Can the children——?
(1) Identify range of sizes from pictures, puppets, flannelgraph, etc. (baby, child, teenager, adult).
(2) Identify sex differentiation during growth, with and without clothes? (boy to man; girl to woman).
(3) Sort out selection of clothes in size order? (baby, child, adult).

* Reproduced by kind permission of the authors.

(4) Contrast short and tall; thin and well-built (fat?) in their own group?
(5) Identify hands of baby, child, adult, old person, from photographs?
(6) Sort out pictures of faces in age order?
(7) —— and in sexes?

1.3 *Feelings*

Can the children——?
(1) Recognise different emotions from pictures? (happy, sad, frightened, angry, loving, lonely, etc.)
(2) Understand what causes these feelings?
(3) Explore in role play (with staff?) what these emotions feel like?

1.4 *Relationships:* self and other people

Do the children——?
(1) Know who helps them?
(2) Realise whom they can help? (other children, family, teachers, etc.)
(3) Know how to express their feeling—through words, gestures, touch, etc.?
(4) Have opportunities to express emotions?
(5) Know how to show friendship?

PART TWO   THE LIFE CYCLE

2.1 *General*

Is the child——?
(1) Familiar with the idea that we are all at some stage between birth and death?
(2) Able to identify people at five stages: baby, child, teenager, adult, old person?
(3) Aware that there are infinite variations from the 'normal'?
(4) Able to understand the concept of growth: i.e., that we grow larger and older?
(5) Aware that growing means changing? (activities, abilities, feelings)

2.2 *Stages in the human life cycle*

Does the child realise that——?
2.2.1 *Babies*
(1) Babies are very dependent: they can do very little for themselves?
(2) Babies need food (breast/bottle)?
(3) Babies need to be kept clean?
(4) Babies need to play (with self, adult, toys)?
(5) Babies need to be loved (cuddling, talking, etc.)?
2.2.2 *Children*
(1) Children can do more things for themselves?

      (2)   They still need food for healthy growth?
      (3)   Children need to be taught to keep themselves clean?
      (4)   Children learn by playing?
      (5)   Children need to love and be loved?

2.2.3 *Teenagers*
      (1)   Teenagers can do many things for themselves and are more independent?
      (2)   —— but they still need parents to love them and help them.
      (3)   Teenagers grow fast and change their shape? (and girls start to have periods)
      (4)   Friends are very important to teenagers?
      (5)   Teenagers enjoy activities with their friends?

2.2.4 *Adults*
      (1)   Adults are fully grown and strong?
      (2)   Adults can look after themselves—independent?
      (3)   Adults often look after other people too?
      (4)   Adults have jobs to do—at work or at home?
      (5)   Adults may live together and set up home together?
      (6)   Adults may have children of their own?
      (7)   Adults take part in many activities (sex differentiation?) e.g. sport, cooking, gardening, DIY, sewing, dancing, etc?
      (8)   Adults need to love and be loved?

2.2.5 *Old People*
      (1)   Everyone grows old in time?
      (2)   Older people are often slower than young people?
      (3)   Older people need family and friends to love?
      (4)   Old people enjoy many activities: talking, meeting people, radio, TV, visiting?
      (5)   Old people are very fond of babies and children?

PART THREE   PERSONAL HYGIENE

3.1 *Washing*

Can the child——?
      (1)   Wash hands and face properly?
      (2)   Use a shower/bath properly, recognising which parts of the body need special care?
      (3)   Clean nails using a nailbrush?
      (4)   Appreciate need for thorough washing?
      (5)   Appreciate need for careful washing if spots occur?
      (6)   Use talcum powder, deodorants, etc., properly?

3.2 *Teeth*

Does the child——?
      (1)   Clean teeth correctly?

196

(2) Know best times to clean teeth?

(3) Have some knowledge of foods that are good and bad for teeth?

3.3 *Hair*

Can the child——?

(1) Wash own hair?

(2) Rinse own hair thoroughly?

(3) Brush/comb own hair?

(4) Dry own hair using towel/hairdryer?

(5) Wash hairbrush/comb?

3.4 *Clothes*

Can the child——?

(1) Understand the need to change clothes regularly?

(2) Use an iron aided/unaided?

(3) Wash simple clothes?

3.5 *Lavatory*

Does the child——?

(1) Use the toilet correctly?

(2) Recognise the need to use toilet?

(3) Wash hands after using toilet?

3.6 *Menstruation*

Does the child——?

(1) Realise when she has started a period in order to ask for help?

(2) Realise when she needs to change a towel?

(3) Manage by herself when reminded?

(4) Manage whole situation unaided?

3.7 *Shaving*

Does the child——?

(1) Know how to shave (using electric/battery razor)?

(2) When to shave?

PART FOUR   GENERAL HEALTH

4.1 *Being ill*

Can the children——?

(1) Identify common complaints: cold, cough, sore throat, joint pain, cut, broken limb?

(2) Cope with basic treatment for each?

Cold	handkerchief, aspirin, rest
Sore throat	keep warm, visit doctor
Joint pain	bandage, perhaps visit doctor
Cuts	sticky plaster

(3) Realise that diseases can be transmitted from one person to another?

(4) Understand the need for adult care during illness?

4.2 *Common cold*

Do the children know——?

(1) How to recognise a handkerchief?

(2) How to blow their noses efficiently?
(3) Where to dispose of soiled handkerchiefs?
(4) How to avoid spreading colds to others?

4.3 *The doctor*
Are the children——?
(1) Able to recognise a doctor (school doctor?) from photographs?
(2) Aware that a doctor is consulted in cases of illness?
(3) Familiar with what happens at a medical examination? (Take temperature, blood pressure, sound chest, etc.).

4.4 *The dentist*
Do the children have a general knowledge of what hapens at a visit to the dentist, including: dental equipment and its use; fillings; injection (local anaesthetic)?

4.5 *Visiting the hospital*
Can the children——?
(1) Identify picture/photograph of local hospital?
(2) Recognise an ambulance?
(3) —— and understand what it is used for?
(4) Understand, in general terms, what happens if someone goes to hospital: e.g., on a day visit (out-patient); staying in a ward; having an operation; medical personnel; visitors?

4.6 *Medicines*
Do the children——?
(1) Recognise a bottle of pills; a tube of ointment; a pack of plasters?
(2) Know how to take medicines; apply ointment; use a plaster?
(3) Recognise the class of treatment called:

      drugs   for internal use
      ointments for external use
      dressings for external use
      injections to be given by medical personnel?

(4) Know that all medicines should be kept safely?
(5) Know never to touch medicines unless given to them by an adult?

PART FIVE   FOOD AND NUTRITION

Does the child——?
(1) Wash his hands before touching food?
(2) Know not to eat dirty food?
(3) Have some knowledge of the term 'special diet' and what this can mean?
(4) Have some knowledge of health foods and those which are harmful when eaten to excess?
(5) Know how to prepare simple and nutritious drinks and snacks?

198

Another comprehensive check list and teaching programme for moderately and severely mentally handicapped individuals may be found in Bender *et al* (1976). The previous chapter in this book describes a hospital based teaching programme for mildly retarded adolescents and adults.

Personal Adjustment Training

Mentally handicapped people who live in institutions often have particular difficulties in maintaining sociosexual identities. They tend to behave less acceptably and to be 'helpless' and 'acquiescent' (Floor and Rosen, 1975; Sigelman *et al*, 1981). Recently in a hospital counselling session I asked a group of mentally handicapped young women to agree or disagree with a series of statements, one of which was "I always do what other people tell me". To this they responded practically with one voice and very pleased with themselves, "Oh, yes, I always do as I'm told. I'm very good, I am". What opportunities there for abuse and exploitation!

Zisfein and Rosen (1973) describe a training programme designed to counteract the low self-concept and esteem and the acquiescence of institutionalised mildly mentally handicapped people. Training manuals were later developed (Elwyn Institutes, 1975).

There are five units:

1. *Self-Evaluation: Identity, self-concept*

   purpose: (a) to improve levels of self regard;
   - (b) to achieve a more realistic match between aspirations and abilities;
   - (c) to increase self-evaluation;
   - (d) to increase awareness of oneself as social stimulus;
   - (e) to improve appearance, grooming, personality traits.

Teaching would include videotape self-confrontation; self ratings.

2. *Acquiescence—Exploitation*

   purpose: to reduce tendency to be acquiescent—submissive to attempts at coercion or exploitation.

This would involve situations such as pill taking; paper signing; financial exploitation.

3. *Assertive Training*

    purpose: to make students less 'helpless', passive and dependent.

Role playing and recording of the tone of voices help people appreciate the relationship between the manner of self-expression and the way in which that person is perceived and treated by others.

4. *Heterosexual Training*

    purpose: (a) to increase repertoires of heterosexual behaviour;
        (b) to decondition anxiety concerning members of opposite sex;
        (c) to increase social awareness;
        (d) to teach coping behaviours for functioning in a bisexual environment.

Again, role playing and modelling on therapist's behaviour, Zisfein and Rosen suggest using a pre-recorded videotape depicting everyday male and female encounters, handled inappropriately and then appropriately.

5. *Independence—Leadership Training*

    purpose: to reduce dependency in problem solving situations.

This gives students opportunities for practice in decision making and problem solving when presented with hypothetical problem situations. For the first, a leader is appointed by the therapist and his/her performance later evaluated by the group; for the next problem no leader is selected. If one emerges naturally the group discusses the difference between the leader's behaviour, and that of group members.

The authors of this paper end by pointing out a number of intrinsic 'underlying ingredients' to their teaching programme. These have relevance to any group counselling and teaching sessions:

A. *Forcefulness of criticism with compassion and support*

Teaching sessions may initiate potentially painful confrontations with personal inadequacies. The therapist has to point out deficits when he sees them, but in such a way that clients are not threatened or antagonised. They must be helped to understand the value of constructive criticism of behaviour.

B. *Recapitulation*

At the end of each teaching session each group member has to recapitulate in his/her own words what has been learned. The therapist must be able to translate concepts (such as assertive behaviour) into terms which have meaning in the lives of the group members.

C. *Therapist involvement*

The therapist must never ask from the client anything that he/she would not do himself. His/her willingness to participate as a group member when appropriate reduces the potential threat and makes it less likely that he/she is seen as distant and judgemental.

D. *Reinforcement of positive self-concept and identity*

The therapist's most fundamental role is as social reinforcer for client responses which are consonant with self-regard and ego development and strength. The therapist's overall approach must convey that each group member is an individual with legitimate ideas, feelings, preferences and biases which he/she has a right to express.

E. *Group members as therapeutic agents*

Mentally handicapped people take each other seriously and can and do offer help to each other. Group dynamics should not be underestimated as powerful instigators of change.

F. *Teaching new behaviours*

'Learning by doing' is very important to retarded people and whenever possible, behaviour is 'practised' within the group as a preparation for the real life occurrence.

Rosen (1970) describes some of the techniques which can be employed to help mentally retarded people to overcome the difficulties they may experience in social and sexual contacts with members of the opposite sex, particularly when they have spent many years in sheltered institutional living, or have been repressed or overprotected by their families.

The prospect of contacts with members of the opposite sex can be frightening to those who have lacked opportunities to learn the necessary social skills. A systematic *desensitisation* programme may decrease the anxiety. This can be achieved by constructing a graduated fear hierarchy, starting with experiences that do not produce fear, for example a group activity like a dance or a party, progressing to individual dating relationships. The client uses deep muscle relaxation and is presented with a structured fantasy representing each level of the hierarchy. Each subsequent step to more frightening situations is only presented when the client reports absence of fear to the preceding fantasy. The client's anxiety is reduced, and he is also acquiring information and suggestions about appropriate behaviour.

After successful desensitisation the client can move on to practise in *programmed heterosexual experiences,* reporting his momentary tension by a simple five-point scale. Again the experiences are graded and a typical progression might be seeing the female therapist at a distance, going to her office, maintaining eye contact, engaging in a predetermined conversation, then a spontaneous conversation, taking a walk with her. After this, the same graded series of behaviours can be done in real situations.

Role playing can be of great value in increasing social skills, enabling clients to practise responses in a non-threatening situation. The therapist can model the desired response and encourage the client to imitate it.

Mentally handicapped people usually do not have access to authoritative sources of information about sexual feelings and behaviour. Jokes, slang expressions, cues may be misunderstood and misinterpreted. The opportunity for frank *talk about sex* with the therapist may in itself reduce anxiety relating to sexuality. Rosen found an absence of *masturbatory activity* in boys with deviant sexual behaviour and had some success in substituting masturbation for inappropriate behaviour.

Problem Behaviour

"If an individual is to be accepted by others, his behaviour must correspond to that which is expected of his age, sex and the culture in which he lives" (Whelan and Speake, 1979).

A major concern of many parents and care staff is the inappropriateness of certain aspects of the behaviour of mentally handicapped people in their care. Almost all human behaviour is learned, not necessarily by means of formal teaching, but by many informal and subtle ways of inference, omission, example and reinforcement. This is very important to bear in mind when we are faced with behaviour which is socially unacceptable—it is not the inevitable result of handicap and we can usually do something to correct it.

202

How can the principles we have been looking at help us alter behaviour for the better?

The first thing called for is a systematic approach, and this is particularly important in the context of sexual behaviours which have all kinds of emotional overtones for parents and care staff. It means an open discussion, a sharing of views, and an agreed plan of teaching and training.

Whelan and Speake (1979) suggest six questions need to be answered:

(1) What is the behaviour which needs to be eliminated?

(2) What cue, event, or situation, seems to trigger it off?

(3) What appears to be rewarding or maintaining the behaviour?

(4) How can this reward be removed?

(5) What positive, incompatible, behaviour should take the place of the behaviour being eliminated?

(6) How is the success of this approach going to be measured and recorded?

They give the following example:

Janet is aged 22 and lives at home with her widowed mother. She is quite attractive and very affectionate—too much so in fact. Mother is beginning to worry at the ease with which she smiles at strangers. When a visitor calls to the house, she readily greets them with an embrace and sometimes a kiss. In most cases, strangers react to this with good humour, tinged with embarrassment. During their frequent conversations, mother has tried discussing this with Janet, but is afraid of damaging her warm personality.

The brief answer to the above questions would be as follows:

Answer 1: Smiling at, embracing, and kissing strangers.

Answer 2: The presence of a stranger, especially a visitor, to her home.

Answer 3: The stranger's smile and good humoured response.

Answer 4: Mother needs some help here from a number of individuals, not known to Janet who agree to help, either by visiting the house, or in some other setting. They should be briefed not to respond too readily when Janet smiles at them (this part of her behaviour we wish to modify, not eliminate entirely). If Janet should step forward to embrace them they should step back, saying "No".

Answer 5: Janet should be taught the appropriate greeting behaviour which should be used after a stranger has been introduced.

She has a good command of language. Her previous embrace should be replaced by a handshake, but only if initiated by the person to whom she has been introduced. Following this correct behaviour, mother should smile at Janet, later remarking that she behaved perfectly.

Answer 6: Mother should keep a simple checklist, to be completed each day. Before commencing her attempt to modify Janet's behaviour, she could record, for each occasion concerned, whether Janet behaved appropriately in the presence of a stranger. She could use a tick, for example, to represent appropriate behaviour and a cross to represent inappropriate behaviour. She may wish, instead of a cross, to use the letters 'S', 'E', 'K', or 'H', to represent a smile, embrace, kiss, or handshake. During the period when mother, with some cooperation from others, is attempting to modify Janet's behaviour, some record should be maintained. The record must be able to show not only the reduction in Janet's inappropriate behaviour, but also the increase in the substituted appropriate behaviour. Scores for successive weeks could be worked out to enable a pattern to be seen more clearly.

Let us look at another example:

Mr. and Mrs. Brown's mentally handicapped 13-year-old son, Colin, has recently discovered how to masturbate and does so frequently, both in the living room and in his bedroom. His two younger brothers, aged eight and ten, are intrigued and impressed. Mrs. Brown was recently very upset and embarrassed when she showed a friend into the living room and Colin was giving a performance to his brothers and another boy. Telling off has had no effect, and Mr. and Mrs. Brown ask for professional advice 'to put a stop to all this'.

In answer to *Question 1* the preliminary discussion may lead to a modification of views. Mrs. Brown particularly wants 'some pills or something' to stop Colin's 'dirty habit' altogether. Mr. Brown is more realistic, and wants Colin to learn 'there's a time and place for everything', but doesn't know how to get that across to Colin. The professional (it could be workshop manager, social worker, community nurse or psychologist) prompts Mrs. Brown to consider how normal masturbation is, particularly among teenage boys. They agree that it is the *public* display that needs to be eliminated.

Question 2: Mr. and Mrs. Brown observed and recorded Colin's activities for a week, and found that two situations frequently preceded Colin masturbating—when his brothers were present and excluded him from a game, discussion or plans; and when his Mum and Dad were much occupied in doing something for or with one of the younger children.

Question 3: Colin had discovered something that he could do, and do well, that his brothers couldn't yet. This was rather rare in his life, as they had overtaken him in many skills. Their attention, admiration, jokes and laughter reward Colin, as does Mum or Dad's switch of attention away from the younger children, even though they get cross with him. This reminds us that even an explicitly sexual behaviour involving the genitals and leading to orgasm, is often engaged in for a whole variety of reasons, only one of which is sexual excitement and physical release.

Question 4: The help of Colin's brothers must be enlisted. They are old enough to understand an explanation that Colin may get himself into trouble outside the home if his behaviour goes unchecked. They should undertake not to encourage Colin, but to ignore his invitations to 'watch me'. If Colin persists they leave the room and Mum or Dad tell him to go to his bedroom.

Question 5: If Colin is present when Mum or Dad are attending to the needs of one of the younger boys, they give Colin verbal reassurance that his turn for attention will come, and ask him to perform some task in the meantime—"I'll just get Tommy his tea before he goes out, and then we can have a look at that new jigsaw of yours. Will you please lay the table, and then I'll be that much quicker?" If Colin masturbates despite this, he is firmly told to go up to his room: "You can do that in your bedroom, but *not* here". The family also decide that they will set aside the hour before the youngest's bedtime for a game of some sort in which everyone can join in.

Question 6: Mr. and Mrs. Brown will need to make a chart to help them record Colin's progress, marking what happened each time Colin began to masturbate in public (see p. 206).

This would be an opportune time for the family to consider the implications of Colin's adolescence, suggesting some kind of sex education and the way in which the household should adapt to the growing adult. For instance, Colin needs more privacy and if they do not already do so, the family should remember to knock before going into his bedroom. Does he have enough opportunities to pursue his own activities and friendships? Does his special school

Day							
1							
2							
3							
4							
5							
6							
7							

√ stopped or went to bedroom

× continued

have a health and sex education programme? Mr. and Mrs. Brown might want some help in choosing suitable sex education books to use with Colin. Mr. Brown will need to show Colin simple hygiene procedures so that he can clean himself after masturbation.

Mitchell *et al* have produced a very helpful manual to aid parents and care staff intervene and modify inappropriate sexual behaviour. They too stress the importance of charting and isolate five important factors:

(1) how often the behaviour occurs—e.g. date, time behaviour starts and stops.

(2) where the behaviour occurs—it may be that the problem behaviour only occurs in one place, and it may be possible to eliminate it by reducing access to this particular location.

(3) what happens just before the behaviour occurs—it may be that a resident starts to masturbate only after he has had an argument, or has failed in some task or activity. The chart might thus show it would be more appropriate to work on the arguing, or on the tasks allocated to the person, than on the sexual behaviour.

(4) what kind of activity the behaviour actually involves—all doing the charting must be clear as to the movements involved, so that they can uniformly record the beginning and end.

(5) what happens immediately after the behaviour occurs—this will usually reveal the 'reward' or 'reinforcement' for the behaviour.

They go on to look separately at problems relating to *place* and problems related to *frequency* with regard to sexual self-stimulation; problems relating to *place* and those relating to the *unacceptability* of certain behaviours in connection with heterosexual and homosexual activity.

Training techniques used with severely and profoundly handicapped people

The literature reports on a number of behaviour modifying techniques which may be used alone, or in conjunction with each other (Lutzker, 1974; Foxx, 1976; Polvinale and Lutzker, 1980; Lombana Durano and Cuvo, 1980). Some of the inappropriate behaviours elminated or greatly reduced by these behaviour modification techniques include exhibitionism, public genital self-stimulation, inappropriate interpersonal sexual behaviour and public disrobing (which of course may not be sexual in intent, but which has a sexual meaning in our society).

A brief explanation of terms may be helpful:

Differential reinforcement of other behaviour (DRO): This may be verbal praise, or verbal praise accompanied by reward such as a sweet or a hug. It is given at the end of a predetermined time interval if the subject is not engaged in the behaviour to be eliminated. Psychologists now usually prefer to employ *differential reinforcement of adaptive behaviour (DRA)* which represents a shift in emphasis from the negative of the subject's problem behaviour to the positive of his adaptive skills. Reinforcement of adaptive behaviour (which may first have to be taught) lessens the likelihood of problem behaviour occurring. DRO raises the question of what the subject will do instead of the problem behaviour, DRA answers it by a forward look at needed skills and concentrates on establishing them, thus preventing a behaviour 'vacuum' into which more problem behaviour can come.

Restitution: This may be physical or social. For example, in the case of stripping, the subject would be required to dress again; or the subject would have to apologise for his behaviour to a set number of people in the room.

Overcorrection: This entails an over-restitution, eg, not only putting clothes back on, but being required to add extra garments and wear them for a set time. It may be accompanied by positive practice such as improving the appearance of others on the ward by brushing hair, straightening clothes, doing up buttons (although one study reported "some of the other residents were resistive or aggressive toward Mary when she assisted them in improving their appearance"! Lombana Durano and Cuvo, 1980).

Time-Out: This may take the form of a set period away from group activities; but it has disadvantages because an individual may use it to engage in an assortment of inappropriate activities that will not be interrupted or discouraged. It must be kept under constant review. Time-out does not necessarily mean the seclusion of the subject, but can refer to a temporary withdrawal of positive reinforcement if the subject is engaging in a problem behaviour.

Ethical Considerations

This chapter has been concerned with ways in which people's adaptive skills can be established and improved. The means that are employed, and indeed the chosen goals themselves, touch upon the ethics of good practice. As the recent *Report on Behaviour Modification* (RCP, RCN and BPS, 1980) points out: ". . . any definition of what behaviour is 'desirable' and what is 'undesirable' always presupposes a value judgment, and may thus be highly controversial" (para. 41). The Report continues:

> When an individual is totally dependent on the responses of others for care, sustenance and even freedom, a generally acceptable definition of desirable behaviour becomes crucial.
>
> It is essential that the demands which are made on patients be appropriately related to their individual needs, abilities and capacity for change, growth and emotional development. At a more fundamental level, it is most important to recognise that all treatments concerned with changing behaviour are based on value judgments. The definition of desirable behaviour is relative. It is likely to vary in accordance with the ideology implicit in the aim of the treatment. For example, the expectation of the staff in Units managing patients simply by custodial care will be very different from those of staff in Units with active rehabilitation programmes. In the same way, the passive, co-operative attitudes appreciated by staff in general medical wards will differ markedly from the autonomy, initiative and responsibility expected of psychiatric patients in 'therapeutic communities'. Great care is needed if the individual's cultural values are to be respected and safeguarded against the unrecognised impositions of the values of the therapist or of the institution. When, for example, is one teaching patients adaptive skills and when is one moulding them into social conformity?
>
> Hence the need arises to consider whether the goals decided upon are

concerned primarily with the needs of the patient or with the convenience of the staff (paras. 43, 44 and 45).

Experience in the United States has shown that without proper safeguards, behaviour modification programmes have on occasion been utilised purely for convenience in administration of an institution. This has led to a series of constitutionally and statutorily induced safeguards against possible abuse. In Britain, the Napsbury Report (DHSS, 1973) revealed instances of what the Report called ". . . a seeming lack of compassion and of respect for the rights of patients" (para 50).

There have been various suggestions and proposals concerning safeguarding the interests of mentally handicapped individuals. No attempt can be made here to cover all the issues involved, but the main elements are briefly discussed.

Environment: Before any attempt is made to modify an individual's behaviour a critical look must be taken at his social and physical environment. As the *Report on Behaviour Modification* (RCP, RCN and BPS, 1980) points out: "There is considerable evidence indicating that an impoverished environment is of itself a cause of disturbed behaviour." Is the individual afforded sufficient opportunities for attention, for interacting with others, for mind-engaging activities, for recreation, for enjoyment? All these are very human requirements, and their absence is likely to contribute significantly to an individual's 'problem behaviour'.

Programmes: Any programme should be based on positive reinforcement, ie on 'rewards', which are over and above the basic and expected standards of care. Only in this context are deprivatory features such as time-out in seclusion permissible. Precise details concerning the total procedure should be written down to guide staff, and these must contain clear instructions as to the extent of deprivatory features, eg the maximum time permitted for seclusion.

Consent: Wherever possible the mentally handicapped person should have explained to him the advantages and disadvantages of the proposed programme and any alternatives, the methods and the goals, and be allowed to make his own decision concerning participation. His relatives should also have the procedure explained to them. If the retarded person is not capable of giving his own consent, his relatives or guardian can take the decision after the points, as outlined above, have been put before them.

Where there are no relatives, special care is required to safeguard the interests of the retarded individual. Various ideas have been put forward, for instance a patient's friend or advocate (appointed from outside the institution or unit), or a review body or committee of some kind.

Responsibility: Most guidelines agree that no one professional or profession should assume the total responsibility for designing and carrying through the behaviour modification programme. The local multi-professional team should discuss and agree programmes, so that decisions concerning the setting of goals and the choosing of methods are made corporately. Such a safeguard would protect mentally handicapped people from over-zealous professionals and inadequately trained ones.

Review: Some formal arrangements should exist whereby the goals, the methods and the results of programmes can be effectively monitored. No programme and no professional should be exempt from ethical scrutiny.

Parents: Of course, parents stand in a different position from staff with regard to formal ethical safeguards. However, in this context it is worth noting that children's interests do not *necessarily* coincide with those of parents. There are many legal examples where a court has distinguished between the interests of a child and those of his parents, but more usually the clashes of interests are of a more subtle nature. For example, parents might pursue the 'interest' of their own peace of mind by keeping their child as close as possible to them. The parents could justify this in terms of it being in the child's best interests to be safeguarded from exploitation and hurt, but from another point of view it might be argued it is *not* in the child's 'interests' to be so cloistered from the world beyond the parental home.

Parents should try and take time to step back a little to think carefully about the targets they wish to set for their child's skills and behaviour. The child (especially an adolescent or adult) should be involved as far as possible in the choice, and have the reward system clearly explained. The whole programme should be geared towards rewarding appropriate behaviour rather than punishing unacceptable responses. Simple but accurate recording allows you to monitor and evaluate progress.

*   *   *   *

210

There are at our disposal a range of approaches and techniques which may be employed to help mentally handicapped people acquire and use the social skills needed to behave normally and to form mutually satisfying interpersonal relationships. The benefits to be gained from improvements accrue as much to parents and care staff as to the retarded individuals themselves.

REFERENCES

Bender, M., Valletutti, P.J. and Bender, R. (1976). *Teaching the Moderately and Severely Handicapped.* Volume 2: Communication, Socialization, Safety and Leisure Time Skills. Baltimore and London: University Park Press.

Cabon, S. and Scott, L. (1980). *A Health Education Check List.* Ickburgh ESNS School, Inner London Education Authority.

Davies, M. (1980). *Sex Education for Slow Learners: A Teaching Aid.* SPOD, The Diorama, 14 Peto Place, London NW1 4DT.

DHSS (1973) *Report of the Professional Investigation into Medical and Nursing Practices on certain wards at Napsbury Hospital, near St. Albans.* London: HMSO.

Fischer, H.L., Krajicek, M.J. and Borthick, W.A. (1974). *Sex Education for the Developmentally Disabled: A Guide for Parents, Teachers and Professionals.* Revised edition. Baltimore: University Park Press.

Floor, L. and Rosen, M. (1975). Investigating the Phenomenon of Helplessness in Mentally Retarded Adults. *Am.J.Ment.Defic. 79,* 5, 565–72.

Foxx, R.M. (1976). The Use of Overcorrection to Eliminate the Public Disrobing (Stripping) of Retarded Women. *Behav.Research and Therapy 14,* 53–61.

Hoffman, M. (undated). *Personal Adjustment Training.* Volume IV: Problem Solving Training. Elwyn, Pennsylvania: Elwyn Institutes.

Lombana Durana, I. and Cuvo, A.J. (1980). A Comparison of Procedures for Decreasing the Public Disrobing of an Institutionalized Profoundly Retarded Woman. *Ment. Retardation 18,* 4, 185–8.

Lutzker, J.R. (1974). Social Reinforcement Control of Exhibitionism in a Profoundly Retarded Adult. *Ment.Retardation 12,* 5, 46–7.

Mitchell, L.K., Doctor, R.M. and Butler, D.C. (undated). *A Manual for Behavioural Intervention on the Sexual Problems of Retarded Individuals in Residential or Home Settings.* Available from Dr L. Mitchell, Department of Counselor Education, California State University, Los Angeles, CA 90032, U.S.A.

Polvinale, R.A. and Lutzker, J.R. (1980). Elimination of Assaultive and Inappropriate Sexual Behavior by Reinforcement and Social Restitution. *Ment. Retardation 18,* 1, 27–30.

Rosen, M. (1970). Conditioning Appropriate Heterosexual Behavior in Mentally and Socially Handicapped Populations. *Training School Bulletin 66,* 172–7.

Rosen, M. and Hoffman, M. (1975). *Personal Adjustment Training.* Volume III: Appropriate Behavior Training. Elwyn, Pennsylvania: Elwyn Institutes.

Rosen, M. and Zisfein, L. (1975). *Personal Adjustment Training.* Volume I: Basic Course; Volume II: Assertive Training. Elwyn, Pennsylvania: Elwyn Institutes.

Royal College of Psychiatrists, Royal College of Nursing and British Psychological Society (1980). *Behaviour Modification.* Report of a Joint Working Party to Formulate Ethical Guidelines for the Conduct of Programmes of Behaviour

211

Modification in the National Health Service. A Consultative Document with suggested Guidelines. London: HMSO.

Sigelman, C.K., Budd, E.C., Spanhel, C.L. and Schoenrock, C.J. (1981). When in Doubt, Say Yes: Acquiescence in Interviews with Mentally Retarded Persons. *Ment. Retardation 19*, 2, 53–8.

Whelan, E. and Speake, B. *Learning to Cope.* Human Horizon Series London: Souvenir Press.

Wish, J.R., McCombs, K.F. and Edmonson, B. (1980). *The Socio-Sexual Knowledge and Attitude Test.* Stoelting Company, 1350 S. Kostner Avenue, Chigago, Ill. 60623, U.S.A.

Zisfein, L. and Rosen, M. (1973). Personal Adjustment Training: A Group Counseling Program for Institutionalized Mentally Retarded Persons. *Ment. Retardation 11*, 4, 16–20.

CHAPTER 10

Sexuality in the Ongoing Lives of Mildly Retarded Adults[1]

Paul Koegel and Robert D. Whittemore

The issue of the sexuality of mentally handicapped adults has been with us ever since mental handicap first emerged as a pressing social concern. From the start, this issue has been a volatile one, sparking strong opinions, equally strong fears, and actions which have had serious consequences for the lives of mentally handicapped people.

Given this long standing concern with sexuality and mental handicap, it is somewhat surprising and certainly unfortunate that the energy devoted to heated polemical debate has not been matched by that expended in empirically-based research. For a long time, empirical research did not seem to be necessary—beliefs regarding the sexuality of this population were so firmly entrenched and seemed so self-evident that to systematically investigate them was seen as belabouring the obvious. Mentally handicapped men were 'known' to be dangerously oversexed, lacking in self-control and, as such, a clear threat to women. Mentally handicapped women, in addition to being promiscuous, amoral and vulnerable, were notoriously fertile and sure to produce feeble-minded offspring. Whether they were viewed as victims or victimisers, it was clear that for their own safety, for the good of society, and for the future of the race, mentally handicapped individuals were best sterilised and encouraged to lead asexual lives in isolation from the community-at-large. From the point of view of delivering services, the implementation of such a policy required answers to administrative, and not research, questions.

Thankfully, the attention directed toward the sexuality of the mentally handicapped today is largely of a different nature. Recent years have seen a general recognition of the right of the mentally handicapped individual to lead as normal a life as possible within his or her community (Wolfensberger, 1972). While the issue of reproductive rights remains a thorny one, many of the old myths

213

have died, and efforts to restrict the sexuality of mentally handi-capped adults have been replaced by a growing commitment to the idea that they, like all people, deserve access to satisfying social and sexual relationships. Professionals involved in providing services to community-based mentally handicapped adults increasingly voice the need for adequate sex education and the provision of settings in which the development of socio-sexual[2] relationships can naturally emerge.

A social policy with such goals *does* demand the answer to a number of research questions and should place a high priority on research. If efforts at education and remediation are to be success-ful, both a rich understanding of what we mean by "sexuality and the mentally handicapped" and an intimate knowledge of the needs and problems of the target population are required. A growing literature has made it clear that in talking about sexuality and mental handicap we are dealing with not one but many issues—educational strategies, psycho-sexual development, the social meaning of having a boyfriend or girlfriend, the mechanics of sex and reproduction, birth control and sterilisation, marriage and parenting. Unfortunately, these issues are all too often considered independently of one another and independently of the perspective of the mentally handicapped themselves. What rarely emerges from the literature (with a few notable exceptions, e.g. Sabagh and Edgerton 1962; Edgerton 1967; Henshel 1972; Mattinson 1975; Craft and Craft 1979) is an appreciation of the way in which these issues are played out in the ongoing lives of these adults. Survey-oriented research efforts (e.g. Hall and Morris 1976; Edmonson *et al* 1979) have told us something about what mentally handicapped individuals know and/or have experienced as far as sex is concerned, though measures are often dependent on caretaker or parent reports (e.g. Mulhern 1975). They have told us little, however, of the less easily identified but more important aspects of sexuality and the mentally handicapped—*their* feelings on a number of these issues and their continuing struggles to understand and experience sexuality within the context of their relationships with others. While difficult to obtain, these kinds of holistic understandings can be a great aid to those providing sex education and counselling, as well as those formulating social policy.

In this chapter, we share both our attempts to reach this kind of understanding based on longitudinal research with a group of mildly

214

retarded adults observed over the course of two and a half years, and our efforts at conceptualising the issues embedded in the larger question of sexuality and mental handicap. By discussing the way in which our research was conducted, our model of socio-sexual adjustment, and the relevant experiences of the members of our research cohort, we hope to contribute to the understanding of an admittedly complex set of issues.

The Community Context of Normalization Study

For a number of years, the Socio-Behavioral Group of the Mental Retardation Research Center (UCLA) has been investigating various aspects of the community adaptation of mildly retarded adults, including the question of what happens to individuals when they are released from institutions to the community (Edgerton 1967; Edgerton and Bercovici 1976) and the quality of life of those individuals living in both small family care homes and larger board and care facilities (Edgerton 1975; Bercovici 1980). In May of 1976, a new project (The Community Context of Normalization Study)[3] was initiated with the aim of exploring the impact of changing attitudes in the delivery of services to mildly retarded adults in their communities. The 'normalization principle' (Wolfensberger, 1972) had by this time become a shibboleth among those providing care and services to retarded individuals. While offering a guiding concept, however, the normalization principle did not put forward a blueprint for the delivery of services, leaving to care providers the task of deciding how the principle should be interpreted and implemented. This project set out to investigate just how this process was taking place, and to document those practices which in fact facilitated and/or hindered the ability of mildly retarded adults to achieve more independent and satisying lives.

To achieve these ends, and to more generally obtain an understanding of the day-to-day lives of mildly retarded adults, a research cohort of 48 individuals was followed for 2½ years. These individuals, ranging in age from 19 to 49 years, had all been labelled mentally retarded by the social services and/or educational delivery system, but were identified by professionals as having the potential for living independently. As such, they represented that segment of the mildly retarded population which stood to gain most from community services influenced by the normalization principle. Some, in fact, were already living on their own; others were living in residential facilities or at home with their parents. Some were married; the majority were single. Many held competitive employment jobs; others worked in sheltered workshops or did not work at all. Table 1 reflects the demographics of this sample as of May 1977; these numbers, however, constantly fluctuated as individual circumstances changed.

Table 1

DEMOGRAPHICS OF THE COMMUNITY CONTEXT
of NORMALIZATION STUDY
(N = 48)

Sex		Employment	
Males	22	Independently Employed	13
Females	26	Workshop	12
		Volunteer	1
Marital Status		None or Unemployed	22
Married	15		
Single	30		
Separated	3	Age	
		18–22	3
		23–27	24
Residential Arrangement		28–32	8
Board and Care	3	33–37	11
Family Care	7	38–42	1
Independent	23	43–47	0
Parents	14*	48–52	1
Residential Programmes	1		

* One lives with in-laws

Generally speaking, intensive qualitative and naturalistic methods were employed as primary means of data collection (see Edgerton and Langness 1978). Each sample member was visited at least twice a month by the same researcher over the course of the research project. These visits, lasting anywhere from one to 12 hours, took place in those settings relevant to the day-to-day lives of sample members, allowing the researcher to become intimately familiar with the places habitually frequented by these individuals and the people with whom they typically interacted. Given the constant and long-term nature of the contract, close relationships quickly developed between researchers and sample members. As researchers became valued and trusted friends, frank and open conversations became possible on topics ranging from work, leisure, feelings about family, counsellors and friends, past events, and hopes for the future, to more private matters such as sexuality and the stigma attached to the mental retardation label. Exposure to the significant others of these individuals and opportunities to interview them more intensively provided additional perspectives on their current and past situations. With time, a large data base, including all that people said and observations of what they actually did yielded a rather full picture of the complex, ever-changing nature of these individuals' lives.

This methodological approach was ideally suited for obtaining information in an area as personal and as sensitive as that of sexuality. Participants were not requested to answer lists of questions asked in meaningless contexts but were rather allowed to introduce the topic when they felt the need or desire to do so. Often, such conversations took place during critical moments, such as the disruption of a relationship with a girlfriend, or after viewing a film that brought back relevant memories. In some cases, discussions about sexuality did not occur until months after research contact had been initiated, and in a few cases, sample members never became sufficiently comfortable with the topic to discuss it openly. By the end of the 2½ years, however, a substantial amount of rich information pertaining to issues of sexuality and social relationships had been gathered.

A Theoretical Model of Socio-Sexuality

To order our data and to clarify the elements that should go into a consideration of sexuality and mental handicap, a theoretical model was developed (Whittemore and Koegel 1978). As noted earlier, many issues have been considered under the rubric of sexuality and the mentally handicapped, ranging from social relationships, to sex itself, to issues of birth control, marriage and parenting. While each of these issues have often been dealt with separately, they are in fact all pieces of a larger whole—they are all aspects, or potential aspects, of paired heterosexual relationships. Because our concern was to both view mentally handicaped adults in a holistic social framework and to show how these varied issues all concurrently feed into the extent to which they are leading satisfying sexual lives, our model was structured in terms of the normative aspects of paired relationships (see Figure 1).

To start, we have recognised that paired relationships in our society are valued for both the pleasure they provide and (usually in their more permanent form) their potential for offspring. We see

217

Fig 1.—A MODEL OF SOCIO-SEXUAL ADJUSTMENT OF MILDLY MENTALLY RETARDED ADULTS

Theoretical Aspects to Paired Relations

Domains of Cognisance, Performance, and Commitment to Pairing

		I. Awareness or knowledge; Cognisance	II. 'Mechanics' or means of performance	III. Attitude or 'commitment' of self
A.	Socially	1. i.e. Individual aware, as a gloss, that paired relationships afford pleasure as a social act.	2. i.e. Individual is aware of, and exercises means by which social contact is established and paired relationships are maintained.	3. i.e. Individual willing to pursue pairing as a social act; actively committed to paired friendship.
B.	Sexually	4. i.e. Individual acquainted with the fact that sexual expressiveness can give pleasure through erogenous zone contact.	5. i.e. Individual aware of how to go about getting and/or giving sexual pleasure.	6. i.e. Individual pursues sexual expression as a desirable aspect of paired relations.
C.	As a social statement	7. i.e. Individual aware that beyond a paired relationship, as in marriage, normative expectations place value on this becoming a father-mother-child triad.	8. i.e. Individual aware that in roles as parents, there are custodial and perhaps other responsibilities; consideration given to the sacrifices for self as well as the changes likely in individual life style.	9. i.e. Individual is committed to having children in spite of potential role revisions and personal sacrifices.
D.	As a reproductive act	10. i.e. Individual recognises the connection between sexual relations and reproduction; though not necessarily nomenclatural, behavioural, understanding of the physiology of intercourse.	11. i.e. Individual aware of existence of birth control technology and its potential utility.	12. i.e. Individual is committed to sexual relations for its reproductive outcome.

Socially

Give pleasure

Sexually

PAIRED RELATIONSHIPS

As a social statement

Do include children

As a reproductive act

pleasure as being social, as in the platonic rewards of paired companionship, represented by Level A; and/or *sexual*, as in the physical/emotional rewards of erogenous activity, represented by Level B. In a parallel way, we interpret the understanding that paired relations do or might *include children* as implying two aspects as well. First, the bearing and care of children can be seen as a social statement (Level C), i.e. proof of normative role assumption. (In this context it is worth noting a recent study which reported that only one per cent of the U.S. population considers marital union without a child to be a desirable state (Silka and Kiesler 1977), an indication of the pressures on mildly retarded adults, who *are* culturally aware, to aspire to become parents.) Second, having children, in addition to its social rewards and implications, involves the *reproductive act* itself (Level D).

Each of these four aspects underlying the consideration, initiation, and maintenance of paired social/sexual ties can be further analysed in terms of three distinct components. An individual may or may not be acquainted with the existence of any one of the four aspects of paired relations (i.e. *general cognisance or awareness*), may or may not be familiar with the *mechanics*, or *means*, of realising that aspect, and finally, may or may not value that aspect in terms of his or her own expectations of paired relationships (i.e. *personal attitude or commitment*). While this last component is perhaps the most difficult to teach to those who do not exhibit it, it may well be the most important of the three. To use Level B as a case in point, where an awareness of the sexual pleasure afforded by paired relations is not accompanied by an understanding of the means by which such pleasure can be achieved, it is fair to assume that a positive attitude or personal commitment to realising sexual gratification will lead to the kind of experimentation which will overcome this ignorance of mechanics. Conversely, a negative attitude toward sexual expression as a desirable aspect of paired relations may forestall sexual involvement even where awareness of its existence and familiarity with 'mechanics' are present.

By dividing each of these four motivational aspects of paired relations into these three distinct components, we are left with twelve cells, each of which earmarks a specific facet of socio-sexual experience. Thus, the model separates the broad area of socio-sexuality into its constituent parts while maintaining them in a holistic framework; while allowing them to be considered separately, it serves as a reminder of how they hang together, and provides the basis for the generation of numerous research questions.

The model, in addition, suggests a working definition of socio-sexual adjustment. Here, adjustment refers less to the positive or negative ratings within any particular cell than it does to the extent of nonconflicting ratings within and between each of the four levels of paired relations. One member of the 'Normalization' project sample, for instance, has negative ratings in both cells 9 and 12, indicating her lack of commitment toward having children and toward having sex for that purpose. This, however, does not indicate poor adjustment. She scores positively in all other cells, indicating a healthy attitude toward both the social and sexual pleasures inherent in paired relations, a knowledge of what goes into raising a child, a decision not to have a child because of the demands involved, and an understanding of how to prevent a pregnancy. Negative ratings, in this case, signal congruence within and between levels, and thus an unproblematic situation. Another woman, engaged to be married, scored positively across levels A, C, and D (signifying her appreciation of the social pleasures of paired relationships, her commitment to having a family after considering the responsibilities and sacrifices involved, and her willingness to engage in sex for that purpose) but showed a great deal of ambivalence across level B. Her confusion over whether sex was indeed pleasurable and her expressed fear of sexual activity dampened her excitement over her impending wedding. While she wanted children, knew the role that sex played in procreation, and was determined to engage in sex at least for that purpose, her ignorance of the pleasurable dynamics of an ongoing sexual relationship placed a great deal of psychological strain on her. Here, negative ratings between levels did in fact indicate a lack of congruence and a real problem.

One major exception must be made to this definition of adjustment as congruence within and across the levels of this model. Congruence, we recognise, can easily be the product of ignorance. Were we to hold fast to our definition, those individuals who remain unaware of even the most basic facts of pleasurable or procreative sexuality but who do not desire children would fall into an adjusted category. Few would outwardly argue the merits of a congruence achieved as a result of ignorance or misinformation, though this is

220

not too far removed from the position presented by those who suggest that educating individuals to non-normative practices can solve the problem of unwanted pregnancy (Johnson 1969, for instance, offers that "some retardates can be taught to consider non-vaginal release the end goal of sexual contact" and that homosexual relationships can eliminate the "hazards of pregnancy"). Informed choice, we believe, lies at the foundation of individual adjustment; within this model, ignorance, regardless of whether it produces congruence, is considered an undesirable state.

Besides organising the varied components that make up the domain of sexuality, suggesting research questions, and implying an operational definition of socio-sexual adjustment, this model suggested a strategy for describing and analysing the data base at hand. Members of the Normalization project sample were assigned ratings (e.g. present or absent) for each of the twelve cells generated by the model. Within each of these cells, identical ratings were grouped together and frequencies compiled. This yielded a general picture of how the sample as a whole was distributed across each of the model's component parts. While providing a general summary of the data, this strategy did not capture the important information embedded in each sample member's individual performance across each of the four levels of the model. For the purpose of considering individual performance across all domains in a more holistic manner, and with the model's interpretation of adjustment in mind, we next examined the pattern of each individual's ratings, grouped like individuals with one another, and analysed the resulting profile clusters for areas of conflict. Taken together, these two strategies revealed a rather detailed portrait of the socio-sexuality of this research sample and the kinds of problems they were experiencing.

In our previous paper (Whittemore and Koegel 1978) we provided a detailed review of the performance of both the sample as a whole by cell and the groupings obtained by clustering individuals who performed similarly across all four levels of the model. While we will not attempt to repeat that review here, we will discuss some of the themes which emerged from these analytical strategies, and illustrate them with the experiences and words of sample members themselves. By allowing them to express in their own words and through their own situations the kinds of problems and needs they have, a better understanding of the population targeted by those

221

concerned with sexuality and mental handicap will hopefully emerge.

Sample Heterogeneity

Perhaps one of the most important realizations to emerge from our attempt to understand the sexuality of persons in our sample is the striking heterogeneity displayed by this group of mildly retarded adults. Much of the literature dealing with sexuality would have us believe that the mentally handicapped can be treated as a uniform group (as in many of the contributions to de la Cruz and LaVeck, 1973). Yet even in a sample restricted to mildly retarded adults alone, individuals manifested remarkably diverse levels of awareness and experience, and highly variable attitudes towards sex, marriage, birth control, and parenting. Brief sketches of a small portion of the sample make this abundantly clear.

To start, there is Faith Castellana.[4] Faith, 28, is married and has two children—a five-year-old son and a baby girl. Her husband, also retarded, is far more handicapped than she, and the responsibility of handling financial matters and running the household falls exclusively on her shoulders. While her husband would love to fill the house with children, Faith is fully aware of the awesome strain that child rearing can entail, and avoided a second pregnancy until she felt ready to handle a new set of demands. She recalled all too well the severe bout of depression she experienced months after her son was born and her aborted suicide attempt at that time. She has since adjusted to the pressures involved in being a mother, and is doing an excellent job of rearing her children. Her formula for success? A child, she believes, must know that there are limits and should be disciplined gently but firmly if those limits are overstepped. But above all, a child should know that he or she is well-loved at all times.

Marge Brainard, 29, is married to an attractive and easy-going construction worker who is not handicapped in any way. They, too, have a five-year-old son, though he has not lived with them since he was eleven months old. At that time, Marge unwittingly bathed him in water that was too hot and burned his bottom. A neighbour, fearing neglect, contacted the authorities, and the court had the child removed from the home, much to the dismay of Marge and her husband. They see their child regularly, however, and expect to regain custody when he reaches the age of six or seven. Meanwhile,

Marge and her husband have no plans for future children and conscientiously use birth control. Marge's only complaint about her sex life is that he husband falls asleep too often on the couch.

Betty and Bobby Gottlieb have been married for four years but have no children. While they sometimes regret their decision, both succumbed to their parents' argument that they would not be able to handle child-rearing (though both disagreed with this assessment), and Bobby had a vasectomy. Their sex life is an active one, however; Bobby, much to his wife's feigned mortification, recalled a Thursday night as "the night it thundered and lighteninged, and the night I got the most I ever got in my life". This comment was hardly surprising given their self-expressed belief that sexual play is one of their most favoured and competently performed activities. Interestingly, Bobby has come to believe that his vasectomy has made it impossible for him to make love with any woman other than Betty.

Jeff and Rhoda Hope, married during the course of research contact (the researcher involved with them served as witness/photographer at their City Hall wedding) only over the strenuous objections of Rhoda's older sister. Of the many fears that loomed in her sister's mind, the fear that Rhoda might become pregnant predominated—in spite of her boycott of all wedding activities, she did manage to page the researcher at City Hall and secure a promise that he would purchase condoms for Jeff. In the face of continued pressure from Rhoda's sister and after discussing the matter with a series of counsellors, Jeff and Rhoda decided that having a child would be too expensive, and that Rhoda, at age 44, was getting a little too old to have a healthy baby. Jeff thus ultimately agreed to a vasectomy. Ironically, had anyone bothered to ask, they would have discovered that Jeff and Rhoda's relationship, before and after marriage, was a platonic one. While remaining a truly devoted couple, sex has simply not been part of their relationship.

Fred Barnett's sex life has been an active one since his release from a state institution some 25 years ago, but he has rarely established intimate social relationships with women. Fred, 50, lives in a somewhat seedy hotel populated by a host of marginal down-and-out individuals. His healthy appreciation of sex has largely been satisfied with prostitutes with whom he has had long-term friendly relationships. One woman in particular has adopted him as a most favoured client, visiting him in his room regularly and charging him ridiculously low prices. Fred often, in fact, refers to her as his girl-friend. Most recently, Fred has faced the unsettling problem of impotence. As Fred laments, "She wants ta, she wants that meat. And I can't even get enough energy to . . . to give it a push, to even get it in. So I says, 'Well, maybe do a little "lollipop work" with it'. You know, she puts a little whipped cream on it and gives it a good lick. She does that for a while and then takes her tongue and keeps goin' down around the side, around the head, tryin' to get a little tickle to it, you know, a little life to it. I get on to her and start to pump a little bit to her and I start gettin' ready to come and it goes soft, goes down, and I just forget it. I says, 'Honey, you've got the five bucks so don't worry about it'." Fred recalls how he used to be able to respond to a woman's advances at a moment's notice, and is visibly disturbed by his new dilemma. Having always prided himself on his sexual prowess, his inability to perform has proved to be quite a blow to his self-esteem.

Jane Benton, a 24-year-old single woman, indicates positive ratings across each level of the model. She often voices her appreciation of the social pleasure inherent in paired relations, pointing to the joys of sharing ideas and experiences with a man. She is very aware of the potential pleasure provided by a sexual relationship, and has indeed experienced such a relationship. She would love to have children, feels she is capable of handling the responsibility, and sees it as a part of her role as a woman. Jane's problem, however, is one of intense sexual frustration. A devout Mormon, she is cognisant of the Church's disapproval of premarital sex, having learned the lesson in a painful manner—she was stripped of her privilege within the Church when it was discovered that she had had sexual relations with her married employer. She received further reinforcement of this lesson when, while seeking reinstatement to her previous status within the Church, her confession to a religious court of Bishops that she had fought strong feelings of wanting her boyfriend to do more than hold her was met with displeasure. Jane is aware that she is sexually frustrated and has been told by a psychiatrist that her inability to derive premarital gratification is placing quite a strain on her. While her body and mind are telling her one thing, however, her Church is demanding the opposite.

Pamela Denson does not share Jane's problem in the least. When her parents died and left her their home, she inherited a perfectly free setting in which to entertain her men friends, usually bus drivers and construction workers she meets at a local donut shop. When she did finally become pregnant, her guardian aunt and uncle interrupted her plans to marry her current boyfriend (the father) and coerced her into both an abortion and a tubal ligation. Pamela is still bitter over this and denies or avoids any mention of the fact that she can no longer have children. Her commitment toward bearing a child is strong; her continued devotion to the memory of her named but unborn baby is revealed in the following quote:

> I still got the baby in my mind once in a while. I used to cry and miss him. . . . The baby's name would have been Jonathan. He'd a' been six months old. This was David Jonathan's baby, the one that was supposed to marry me. He came home one day and says, "I thought you were going to have a baby." And I says, "Yeah, my s.o.b. aunt and uncle made me have an abortion." And he says, "Aren't we gonna have the baby?" And I says, "No, they made me give it up." He was so upset about it and that was when he left me. . . .

Katy Chalmers' first experience with sex was when an older half-brother raped her, an experience she has not easily forgotten. While Katy desperately wants to get married, immediately falls in love when any eligible man expresses interest in her, and assumes a new vivacity and charm whenever she believes she has resolved her quest for a permanent relationship, she continues to remain ambivalent regarding sex. Thus, while she willingly, if reluctantly, accompanied her boyfried to a local motel on a weekly basis (her family-care facility was not a setting in which love-making was condoned), these jaunts increasingly disturbed her, and she broke up with her boyfriend in a very sudden and abrupt manner. She confessed that she hated going to the motel, not only because it was a waste of money that should be saved for marriage, or because it meant lying to her caretaker, but because she was not interested in sex. She realised that sex was a part of marriage and was willing to play along when the time came. But she received no pleasure from it herself and was surprised by a researcher's comment that it was something a woman might enjoy. She did want children, and would have gladly tolerated sex toward that end; unfortunately, her father forced her to undergo a tubal ligation. Like many parents, he led her to believe, contrary to adoption agency policy, that if she wanted children in the future, she could adopt.

225

Kevin Knowles, on the other hand, is convinced that he doesn't want children—he sees them as being pesty little creatures who are more trouble than they are worth. He would love to have a girlfriend, but confesses that he does not know how to go about meeting and dating the kind of woman with whom he would want to be seen. Kevin accepts that he is mildly handicapped, but prefers not to associate with other handicapped individuals. He feels intimidated by non-handicapped women, however, and strongly suspects that his chances of holding the interest of such women are slim. Thus he remains a social isolate, his only sexual activity being masturbation. A brief infatuation with pornographic movies left him somewhat ambivalent about sexual expression; the seedy antics of the characters in the film shocked him and left him temporarily convinced that abstinence might be the most well-advised choice.

For Charley Norton, aged 23 and living in a family care facility, any mention of sex is the cause of intense embarrassment. He is fully aware of sex, reproduction and birth control, having listened to the explanations of his mother and a teacher at the state institution where he spent his entire adolescence, but tries to avoid any discussion of these matters. He has dated the same woman for some three years, and seems happy with her despite his repeated complaints about her shrewish nature. They spend a good deal of time together, but do not have a chance to spend that much time alone in either his family care home or her parent's home. Charlie has claimed not to be interested in sex on some occasions; on other occasions he has intimated that he and his girlfriend have engaged in some exploratory experimentation. In either event, a drawerful of magazines filled with pictures of naked women belies his stated disinterest. What he lacks are the same opportunities for the expression of his interest which are open to other men of his age.

Hal Lorne, at age 36, lives an even more restricted life. He, too, lives in a small family-care home with four co-residents whose lives are strictly controlled by a woman they all refer to as 'Mom'. He leaves the house in the morning for the sheltered workshop along with his housemates, returns home in the afternoon, and remains in the house with the exception of weekend jaunts, also in the company of his house-mates. He spends much of his time writing short stories and expresses no interest in either women, sex, marriage, or children. While he has led us to believe that his past life has included social and sexual experience with women, whatever need he had for female companionship has long been represssed as he has adjusted himself to the reality of his current situation.

Though thirty-four and completely committed to the social pleasures derived from his relationships with girlfriends, Johnny Compton, who lives with his parents, remains totally ignorant of even the most rudimentary aspects of sexuality. An affable and mannerly gentleman, he has had no trouble finding girlfriends. But he gives no indication to researcher, parents, or even other handicapped friends, that he has any awareness of sex or the physiology of reproduction whatsoever. To Johnny, this ignorance does not seem to be a problem at all. But a close friend of his wonders how he can ever have a normal marital relationship with a woman given the extreme state of his naivete.

These sketches should make it clear, then, that a wide range of experience and attitude characterises this research cohort and, by implication, mentally handicapped individuals as a group. One cannot generalise from the retarded population as a whole to any one particular individual in a domain of behaviour as extraordinarily complex as socio-sexuality. One cannot say of this population that *all* need sex education, or that *all* need birth control training or intervention, or that *all* are incapable of raising children successfully. One cannot assume that all are reconciled to childless marriages, that all have opportunities to pursue heterosexual friendship, or that all even value sexual relationships. Rather, this is a population whose diversity certainly matches, and probably supersedes, that of any comparable population of normal individuals. Their dramatically differing experiences remind us that each individual is unique, and must be treated as such.

Diverging Understandings of Social and Sexual Pleasure

With this sample heterogeneity in mind, we turn to some of the incongruities which emerged as being relevant to differing groups of sample members once analysis of the data in terms of the model took place. First of all, the uniformity with which project members responded across Level A of the model is striking, and signals their wholesale appreciation of the social pleasure involved in paired relations. Given this appreciation and the understanding of how to realise it, it is important to note that at least a third of the same individuals failed in Level B to rate equally positively on the sexual pleasure such relationships potentially afford. These individuals often evinced no understanding that sexual pleasure between couples could exist, and at best were aware of this in some hazy way but rejected the notion in terms of their own experience. It would seem that classrooms, work settings, social groups, and other organised leisure activities provide mildly retarded individuals with opportunities to explore the cultural value placed on male-female social ties. But to assume that outside such settings social companionship can or will evolve into sexual partnership is, for at least this third of our sample, an ill-conceived notion. There is no reason to believe that mild retardation, as a handicapping condition, should in any way affect a person's ability to perform sexually. This leads us to hazard that the problems of these individuals are most likely related to the values and practices of those significant others involved in their ongoing socio-sexual socialisiation.

The issue of socio-sexual socialisiation brings to the fore a second, related theme. An impressively larger number of participants in the study are aware of the physiology of reproduction (Cell #10) and even the technology of birth control (Cell #11) than are aware of the existence or mechanics of pleasure (Cells # 4 and 5) potentially involved in sexual expressivity. Educational efforts, both formally from professionals and informally from parents and peers, seem to have had greater success in imparting the more biological aspects of heterosexual pairing than the more dynamic, pleasurable dimension. In that parents and professionals so often end up discouraging mildly retarded individuals from parenting, it is ironic that they are successfully teaching the one aspect of sexuality they then discourage their charges from exploring.

The case of John Hamlin, 25, illustrates both of these themes and provides, in addition, dramatic evidence of the pay-off which justifies the time-consuming and painstaking methodology employed in this study. Fond of relating and responding to jokes requiring an intimate awareness of sexual innuendo, John also readily ogles the anatomy of attractive women and refers casually to three past relationships with girlfriends. Given this evident appreciation and knowledge of sexuality, it came as quite a shock when John revealed the actual state of his sexual knowledge to his researcher some five months into their relationship. In a conversation initiated by his characteristic delivery of a sex-related joke, John was urged by the researcher to discuss how he had first learned about sex. As the conversation proceeded, it rapidly became clear that John's apparent sophistication was a self-created veneer masking an underlying ignorance and confusion. John was aware that male-female genital contact was involved in the creation of children, having learned of such matters from his father and in a similar biologically-oriented discussion in school. He was completely and utterly baffled, however, by the suggestion that in addition to producing children, sex served as an inherently pleasurable exercise; he had in no way linked paired sexual activity in any form (kissing, petting or making love) with the pleasurable release he experienced in solitary masturbation. Behaviour that made complete sense to others was thus an enigma to him. His struggles to understand either the motivations of his girlfriend in having engaged in mutual masturbation with a previous boyfriend, the concept of sexual fantasy, or even the bedroom scenes in movies all proved hopelessly futile.

In spite of his confusion, John had come to realise through the constant good-natured ribbing of his co-workers that sexual performance is an expected component of adult life. Afraid of exhibiting his naked form before a woman, unaware of foreplay or that sexual intercourse consists of something more than simply inserting a limp penis into the gaping hole he assumed female genitalia to be, and convinced that the effort would reward him with nothing but anxiety, John could only answer that he 'wasn't ready'. But he worried that his reluctance to engage in sex would interfere with his chances of achieving desired marital union. Upon hearing that most women did indeed enjoy sex and assumed sexual activity to be a natural component of paired relations, John figured that a woman who didn't want, or even better, couldn't have children would be the only solution of his problem. He reasoned that a woman uninterested in the possibility of childbirth would in no way desire sex, again betraying his basic confusion.

For John, the provision of education and appropriate settings for experimentation may be late. Indeed, the attempts of the researcher to cope with John's confusion and the questions it generated failed for lack of a foundation on which to build an understanding of the pleasurable aspects of sexuality. Amazingly, he has reached the age of twenty-five and achieved a fair degree of social sophistication with no realisation that for others, making love is a valued experience in its own right. In the final analysis, while he can envision making love for procreative purposes, his attitudes toward and understandings of sexual activity militate against the realisation not only of this reproductive goal but also of an opportunity to healthy and long-lasting heterosexual friendship.

Parenting and Sterilization

As we have tried to imply in our model, it is impossible to consider sexual expression and the mentally handicapped without at the same time considering the issue of reproduction. Parents and cohort members alike have offered substantial evidence that these two issues are inextricably linked: parents often express fears that their retarded sons and daughters will bear children which they will be unable to raise, and therefore intervene in their children's relationships so as to minimise this possibility; retarded adults, on the other hand, often express their recognition that it is 'normal' to get married, and that marriages typically lead to children.

Again, heterogeneity is the rule when it comes to attitudes toward and experience with parenting among sample members. Some forty percent of the sample have indicated a commitment to the idea of having children. The comment one woman made (directed toward the objections voiced by her parents over the possibility of her and her boyfriend eventually having a child) is not atypical: "We went to see Don, a friend of ours, last night who is working very hard. His wife is supposed to have a baby the end of January. Now what I'm trying to say, everybody we know is having kids. We want to have a baby, too, and we can't have one. I don't think it's fair!" On the other hand, the remaining sixty percent of the sample have either not mentioned children, have expresssed ambivalence over the idea of having children, or have rejected the idea after having considered it. One woman, who is afraid that her epilepsy will interfere with her ability to parent, has said, "I'd like to have kids but I just can't take care of them like I should. I know I won't have any kids. I don't want any because I am afraid. If I have a seizure and I have a baby, I don't want that. I'll just take care of my sister's kids."

Likewise, heterogeneity characterises those five sample members who are parents. Faith and Marge have been mentioned earlier as examples of successful and unsuccessful parents. Marilyn and Rich Williams offer a more complicated case. Marilyn had her first child during the course of research contact and proved to be a caring and competent mother. Rich, however, was disappointed that the baby was not a boy and vowed that they would try again until they got it 'right', this in spite of the fact that he took no responsibility for either caretaking or holding a job. Three years and two more baby girls later, Marilyn convinced him that she could not continue having a baby a year to satisfy his whim, and Rich had a vasectomy. Meanwhile, she is having a great deal of difficulty coping with the strain of running a household and raising three children, all under the age of five. Finally, Peg Ingham, like Marge, had her child taken from her because of negligence—she and her ex-husband went out for the evening and left their infant at home alone.

Our data on parenting experience, admittedly limited, does no more than support the conclusion suggested by the sketchy literature on this topic (e.g. Mickelson 1947; Mattinson 1975; Andron and Goldberg 1978; Craft and Craft 1979) that some retarded individuals will parent successfully while others will not. Our data on *attitudes* towards parenting, however, suggest a potential area of conflict in the socio-sexual adjustment of a significant segment of this population. While many individuals have at least temporarily rejected the idea of having children, a good many see parenthood as a desirable social role. Those who would exert influence over them, however, often question their ability to assume this role, and are often prepared to take steps to prevent parenthood.

This conflict is perhaps most clearly embodied in those individuals (15% of the sample) who are committed to the role of parenting but who cannot have children because they or their spouses have been surgically sterilized. (In total, approximately 30% of the sample have been sterilized themselves or have a sterilized spouse.) In all of these cases, sterilization, as required by law, was voluntary. A careful look at the process by which these individuals came to agree to an operation (see Haas 1979) reveals, nevertheless, that a signature on a consent form does not ensure that a decision has been reached after careful and independent consideration. In fact, individuals in our sample have been coerced into obtaining surgery as a precondition to marriage or living together, have been sterilized as part of an abortion without full information having been provided, and have signed consent forms for an operation in times of stress and personal instability. We mention this not to engage in the polemics of the sterilization issue, though such a debate may well be timely. Rather, we do so because the experiences of our sample population in this regard suggest that long-term difficulties in adjustment to such permanent sterilization procedures bear directly on other facets of socio-sexual adjustment. The way in which this can take place is exemplified by the experiences of Chrissy Cole and Billy Scheff.

Chrissy and Billy met at the house of a mutual friend and began dating soon thereafter. Neither came to the other totally inexperienced. In fact, Chrissy had been married before and was, at the outset of her relationship with Bill, taking birth control pills. Chrissy, however, was the first woman with whom Billy had made love.

Some years into their relationship, Chrissy began putting on weight distributed in a peculiar enough manner to motivate a comment from a perceptive aunt that she 'looked funny'. A doctor's visit confirmed that Chrissy was indeed five months pregnant. Chrissy offers that her condition came as a complete surprise to her. Others are reasonably sure that she had purposely discontinued her use of the pill and that her pregnancy was not an accidental occurrence.

While it was crystal clear to Chrissy's mother that a therapeutic abortion was the only solution to this unfortunate problem, Chrissy saw her condition as neither unfortunate nor a problem. In her resolve to keep her unborn child (whose movement she had already felt) she was supported by her brother, her psychiatrist, and even Billy's mother. Her mother, however, was convinced that Chrissy could not successfully manage parenting and adamantly insisted that she would have to abort the child. Her resolve proved stronger than Chrissy's, and unhappy but drained by the incessant arguing, Chrissy acquiesced to her demand.

When Chrissy and Bill decided to move into an apartment together, Chrissy's mother prevailed once again. As a precondition of their cohabitation, Billy was told that he would have to have a vasectomy. The idea was not pleasing to him at all, but at the time his desire to be with Chrissy clouded considerations of future progeny. A vasectomy was performed soon after the abortion, and the two of them established a home together, assuming the roles of husband and wife in spirit, if not in law. Billy became quite embittered, prone to such statements as: "Chrissy's mother ruined me by forcing the vasectomy on me." Chrissy, on the other hand, alternately blamed Billy and her mother for the loss of her unborn child, and continued to overtly relate future happiness to the role of motherhood. "All I want," she said, "is to be happy and have my baby." This was quite threatening to Billy, who was aware that he couldn't fill the need she consistently reiterated. His only recourse was to try to convince Chrissy that she didn't want what she insisted she did want.

As time passed, it became increasingly clear that these concerns were translating themselves into negative consequences for Chrissy and Billy's sexual relationship. Initially, indirect clues served as evidence: single day beds in the living room took the place of the large double bed in the bedroom, and oblique reference was made to the fact that while they were living together, they were not necessarily sleeping together. Any physical affectionate overture on Billy's part was coldly rebuffed by Chrissy. Finally, the issue surfaced. First, Chrissy, in Billy's absence, confessed that she found any physical contact with Billy distasteful, and that all she thought about when Billy touched her was "the baby which they took from me. I think about holding the baby and rocking and playing with it." Later, Billy also revealed his belief that his vasectomy and their current inability to have a child was at the root of their sexual problems, and he and Chrissy frankly discussed their reasons for wanting to get the vasectomy reversed.

Billy: "We were going together for three months. When I first met her, she wouldn't leave my body alone. She wanted to have sex every night. . . . Since I had this vasectomy, she doesn't have that kind of feeling."

Chrissy: "Every time he wants to do anything, I see myself sitting in a rocking chair with the baby."

Billy: "Every time I make love to her, the thing goes in her head. Am I going to have a baby this time or never? That's why I'm going to have it [the vasectomy reversal] done. Because I want to have her the way she was when I first met her. And she would be the way when I first met her. . . . She wouldn't stop having sex. She would just go all night. If I had it done she would be exactly the same way as when I first met her. I'll never forgive her parents. Next time, if we want a kid, we're gonna have one."

With the exciting plans of marriage and a child at hand, a dramatic change took place in the nature of Billy and Chrissy's relationship. More than receptive to Billy's affectionate overtures, Chrissy herself initiated them and spoke of their future with no hint of the uncertainty that had previously infused her plans. But as it appeared that Medi-Cal was not going to cover the anticipated operation, and that the prohibitive cost of a reversal more than surpassed their financial resources, Chrissy once again displayed signs of unrest and dissatisfaction. Her discovery that her cousin was pregnant depressed her, and she jokingly noted that she was tempted to "go out and get pregnant by anyone." Her suspicious behaviour made Billy rightly believe that she was secretly seeing a former boyfriend, and this placed yet a larger strain on their overly taxed relationship. It was not at all long after the realization that a reversal was not possible that their relationship came to a stormy end. To this day Billy's and his mother's bitterness continues over his own infertility and the fact that Chrissy was left free to find a mate and have a child.

Problematic Partners

The themes and longer case studies presented thus far have focussed largely on major issues in socio-sexual adjustment as revealed by individuals who exhibit incongruent ratings within the model presented above. This is not to say that these individuals who consistently display congruent performance across and between the levels of the model live problem-free lives as far as sexuality is concerned. While holistic, the model itself can tell us only so much. Because it considers the individual independent of those with whom he or she interacts (parents, friends, lovers), it fails to account for the dynamics of many individuals' experiences. Individuals like Jane (see page 224) may be perfectly adjusted in terms of the parameters of the model but be frustrated by parents, religious doctrines, etc. in their attempts to gratify themselves sexually, or to have the children they want. An equally pressing problem lies in the fact that adjusted individuals most often choose mates who are also developmentally disabled. We have seen that this group, as a whole, exhibits relatively high rates of problematic social/sexual behaviour. The chance is thus increased that 'adjusted' individuals will face difficulties because of the problems of their 'nonadjusted' partners. The frustrating and upsetting nature of Rachel Grant's experience more than demonstrates this.

For Rachel, a vibrant, healthy woman of twenty-one, a four-year partnership with her boyfriend, Rob, has offered both joys and frustrations. She admits that her parents' description of Rob as a loafer, a malcontent, and a depressive are largely accurate. Even so, she continues to be intrigued by his ability to attract her and feels strongly that her future happiness rests on the continuation of their relationship. Marriage and children are desired goals for her, but only if realised with Rob. No other young men interest her, she claims.

Rachel's problems stem from a lag between her appreciation of her sexual needs and feelings, and Rob's awareness of his. She has frequently discussed her self-recognised sexuality, and has readily confessed to dreams of kissing "a real nice muscley guy"; thoughts of more serious sexual encounters enter her daytime fantasies as she eyes attractive men that pass her way. While Rachel is sometimes confused by the strength of her feelings ("It's not normal for girls to want to hop into bed with every Tom, Dick, and Harry") she accepts them and understands the social mores channelling the expression of them.

Though Rachel offers that "there is just something in me that I just want to do it with really cute guys", she overtly acknowledges that she would love nothing more than to be able to satisfy her longings with Rob alone. It is his failure to respond to her needs, and her consequent frustration, that sets her mind wandering toward fantasised relationships with other men. For Rob and Rachel, there are ample opportunities for sexual activity in that Rob has his own apartment. But, as Rachel laments, "Nothing happens. Nothing ever happens when me and him are together. He doesn't get fresh or nothing. He's a shy person. He has his best friend. I don't know what's the matter but I think they're a little bit gay . . . I don't know. I'm really confused. I mean, I want him so bad!"

Rachel's frustrations have indeed driven her to other men. For a few months she dated an aggressive, attentive young man who soon made his serious social and sexual intentions known. Rachel, in fact, cared for and "almost went all the way with this guy." "I don't know," she said. "It was weird. I needed Rob so bad that I just wanted to have sex with somebody. I don't know why." While confessing that she was sorely tempted on one occasion to allow their explicit petting to reach its natural end, her friend respected her ultimate decision to, at least for the moment, restrain herself.

Despite her new boyfriend's devotion to her, for Rachel there was really no question that she continued to love Rob, and she soon returned to him, as well as the problems she had faced in their relationship. His continued emotional hold on her is something she

235

finds difficult to explain. Poignantly, she discusses her current dilemma: "I like to go with him. I like to be with him. Something about him. I really don't know why I'm so thrilled over him. It's a weird thing. In my eyes, he's cute, but that's not the only thing I dig. Maybe it's his body. He's not so muscley or anything but just the way he is . . . I don't know why. He touches me and I go into orbit. I'm so confused. It hurts. You want to be in love at the same time as the other person. Loving alone is not helpful."

Conclusion

In this chapter, then, we have pursued a number of ends. To start, we have portrayed the extreme diversity of attitude and experience displayed by mildly retarded individuals with regard to sexuality-related issues. These individuals do share a social label, but to treat them as a homogeneous group is to ignore the marked differences in their early and continuing socialization experiences, their present life circumstances, and their overall appreciation of their sexual/reproductive potential. Some are sexually sophisticated; others are shockingly naive. Some can use temporary means of birth control responsibly; others are not even aware of how to prevent conception. Some see marriage and/or parenting as desired ends; others shy away from them. The heterogeneity of this population is perhaps its single most striking feature.

Through our model of socio-sexual adjustment, and our discussion of themes and case material as they relate to the model, we have also stressed the folly of trying to treat various aspects of sexuality as separate and independent entities. The social, erotic, and reproductive aspects of paired relationships are all inextricably linked; a problem in one may very well affect the others. Bitterness over restrictions on reproductive potential can spill over into the healthy functioning of a relationship both sexually and interpersonally. Confusion over the meaning of erotic activity can reduce one's chance of establishing and maintaining a desired relationship. Identification of sex solely in terms of its reproductive function can result in complete puzzlement over why people sometimes behave as they do, in day-to-day lives as well as in the media.

While we have not stressed this point, another crucial lesson that emerges from our research is that the lives of mildly retarded people *do* change over time, often radically and unpredictably. One woman, for example, who lived with her parents during the period of research contact, showed no understanding of the mechanics of sex in either its pleasurable or reproductive sense. Her life and interests were so patterned, at that time, that the researcher assigned to her had jokingly dubbed her "boring Barbara". Shortly after the end of research contact[5], however, she entered an independent living training programme, fell in love, came to suspect that she was pregnant, eloped, and found that she was not pregnant shortly thereafter. She and her husband, who have decided not to have children, have since then had no lapses in their use of contraception. Both have graduated from the programme, are living in their own apartment, and are quite happy. Chrissy Cole did marry a former boyfriend, did ultimately have a child, and has proved to be a competent mother. Johnny Compton, in spite of continued sexual ignorance, is currently engaged and preparing to move out of his parents' house in anticipation of his wedding. Marge Brainard's husband found another woman, leaving her unable to look after herself independently and with reduced opportunities to maintain contact with their son. Changes, it becomes clear, can solve old problems but can also create new ones.

All of these points carry implications for the work of sex educators and counsellors. This population's heterogeneity, first of all, makes it clear that not every mildly retarded adult will need sex education and counselling, and that those who do will likely exhibit varying and unique problems. Each person must thus be dealt with independently of the pre-conceptions that all too often attach themselves to those with a handicapped label; each deserves to be treated as an individual.

In a similar vein, it must be recognized that an individual's needs and problems will change over time as his or her circumstances change. The individual we see today may be totally different five years hence: the irresponsible and promiscuous twenty year old may settle into a more judicious twenty-five year old; the totally naive young adult may naturally arrive at a full appreciation of sexuality much later with the advent of a new relationship. More than sensitizing sex educators and counsellors to the changes their clients may undergo, this realization suggests the danger of seeking permanent solutions to what may be temporary problems. Individuals who currently voice no objection to sterilization, for

237

instance, may later regret relinquishing their reproductive potential for any number of reasons: meeting a mate who is committed to having, and capable of rearing, children; personal changes in attitude towards parenting; advances in competence and self-image which open doors that had previously appeared closed. Temporary measures are better tailored to the unpredictability of lives in process, and may save individuals the potential pain of future conflicts.

Our emphasis on the inter-connected nature of social, erotic and reproductive aspects of sexuality places yet other burdens on sex educators. By and large, sample members suggested that sex education programmes to which they were exposed dealt with the "facts of life"—the mechanics of sexual intercourse, the physiology of reproduction, and methods of contraception. We rarely heard sample members speak of sex education programmes which highlighted the continuing role of sexuality in ongoing relationships, though it is within this area that cohort members displayed the most ignorance. Education as to mechanics and the provision of social settings in which handicapped men and women can meet is often not enough. Many mentally handicapped individuals have led isolated and restricted lives; some have been denied access to the informal processes by which non-handicapped individuals arrive at understandings of human sexuality. For these individuals, an attempt must be made to expand our concept of sex education to include, in addition to mechanics and reproduction, an effort to communicate the social and pleasurable dynamics of sexuality, and an understanding of the place of sex in the social life of most adults. As for counsellors, this holistic view of sexuality as being many interconnected facets suggests the need for careful consideration of how one area can affect others, particularly when it comes to the admittedly complex issue of reproductive rights.

We realize that we have raised more questions than we have answered, and thus close with a reminder of the important role to be played by research in learning more about sexuality and mental handicap. There is much that we do not understand. We do not know enough about the socialization experiences of retarded children and adults to appreciate how it is that their knowledge of and commitment to sex may have been inhibited. We do not know enough about how non-handicapped children and adolescents informally come to learn the subtle nuances which, in addition to more basic information, comprise a complete understanding of human sexuality. We do not know how to best approximate this informal learning process in formal educational settings. We do not know enough about the long-term consequences of sterilization, or the characteristics which separate those retarded adults who will parent adequately from those who will not—indeed, we know far too little about what comprises adequate parenting. While not easy to obtain, answers to these questions and to a myriad of others have much to contribute to efforts aimed at ensuring that mentally handicapped individuals most fully achieve their potential as adults within their communities.

NOTES

(1) The research for, and preparation of, this chapter was made possible by the Mental Retardation Research Center, UCLA (USPHS Grant HD-04612-05) and by the Community Context of Normalization Study (NICHD Grant HD-09474-02). We gratefully acknowledge the contributions of Laurel Ashley, Lorel Cornman, Candy Fox-Henning and Patti Hartmann to the collection of data, and the helpful comments of Robert B. Edgerton and Sharon Sabsay during the writing of this chapter.
(2) While cumbersome, we use the term "socio-sexual" as opposed to "sexual" to stress the fact that we are dealing with not only sexual activity itself but the social relationships in which sexual activity is typically pursued.
(3) Robert E. Edgerton, Principal Investigator, NICHD Grant No. HD-09474-02.
(4) Pseudonyms have been used to protect the identity of all sample members. These sketches, in addition, are based on information that existed as of 1978. The life circumstances of many of these individuals have changed since then.
(5) While the Normalization study ended in 1978 after thirty months of research contact, a periodic contact has been maintained with a good many of these individuals since that time. Some of them are currently members of a sample being followed as part of a five year study of the community adaptation of mildly retarded adults.

REFERENCES

Andron, L. and Goldberg, I. (1978). *Motherhood: What it is like if you are poor and developmentally disabled.* Paper presented at the 102nd Annual Convention of the American Association of Mental Deficiency, Denver.

Bercovici, S. M. (1980). *The Deinstitutionalization of the Retarded: Community Management of a Marginal Population.* Unpublished doctoral dissertation, University of California, Los Angeles.

Craft, A. and Craft M. (1979). *Handicapped Married Couples.* London: Routledge and Kegan Paul.

de la Cruz, F.F. and LaVeck, G.D. (eds) (1973). *Human Sexuality and the Mentally Retarded.* New York: Brunner/Mazel.

Edgerton, R.B. (1967). *The Cloak of Competence.* Berkeley: University of California Press.

Edgerton R.B. (1975). Issues relating to the quality of life among mentally retarded persons. In: Begab, M.J. and Richardson, S.A. (eds) *The Mentally*

239

Retarded and Society: A Social Science Perspective. Baltimore: University Park Press.

Edgerton, R.B. and Bercovici, S.M. (1976). The cloak of competence: Years later. *Am.J.Ment. Defic. 80,* 485–97.

Edgerton, R.B. and Langness, L.L. (1978). Observing mentally retarded persons in community settings: An anthropological perspective. In: Sackett, G.P. (ed). *Observing Behavior, Vol. I: Theory and Applications in Mental Retardation.* Baltimore: University Park Press.

Edmonson, B., McCombs, K. and Wish J. (1979). What retarded adults believe about sex. *Am.J.Ment. Defic. 84,* 11–18.

Haas, L.M. (1979). *The mentally retarded and the social context of fertility control.* Working paper No. 9, Socio-Behavioral Group, Mental Retardation Research Center, School of Medicine, University of California, Los Angeles.

Hall, J.E. and Morris, H.L. (1976). Sexual knowledge and attitudes of mentally retarded adolescents. *Am.J.Ment. Defic. 80,* 382–87.

Henshel, A.M. (1972). *The Forgotten Ones.* Austin: University of Texas Press.

Johnson, W.R. (1969). Sex education and the mentally retarded. *J.Sex Research, 5,* 179–85.

Mattinson, J. (1975). *Marriage and Mental Handicap.* London: Institute of Marital Studies, Tavistock Institute of Human Relations (2nd edition).

Mickelson, P. (1947). The feebleminded parent: A study of 90 family cases. *Am.J.Ment. Defic. 51,* 644-53.

Mulhern, T.J. (1975). Survey of reported sexual behavior and policies characterizing residential facilities for retarded citizens. *Am.J.Ment. Defic. 79,* 670–73.

Sabagh, G. and Edgerton, R.B. (19662). Sterilized mental defectives look at eugenic sterilization. *Eugenics Quarterly 9,* 213–22.

Silka, L. and Kiesler, S. (1977). Couples who choose to remain childless. *Family Planning Perspectives 9,* 16–25.

Whittemore, R.D. and Koegel, P. (1978). *Loving alone is not helpful: Sexuality and social context among the mildly retarded.* Working Paper No. 7, Socio-Behavioral Group, Mental Retardation Research Center, School of Medicine, University of California, Los Angeles.

Wolfensberger, W. (1972). *The Principle of Normalization in Human Services.* Toronto: National Institute on Mental Retardation.

CHAPTER 11

Birth Control Techniques and Counselling for a Mentally Handicapped Population

Rona MacLean

Introduction

Trends in the pattern of care for the mentally handicapped continue to be away from segregated custodial care in large institutions and towards community living. Hostels are at last becoming available and in some areas Group Homes are already well established. The ability of mentally handicapped people to live successfully in the community is now recognised. In future, only a minority will require hospital care—the severely multiply handicapped, and the mildly handicapped who, because of behavioural problems which have brought them into conflict with society, need a period of treatment and training in a more intensively supervised setting. One consequence of this liberalisation has been the greatly increased oportunities for developing heterosexual relationships which may in their turn result in the risk of an unwanted pregnancy.

These welcome changes in the pattern of care bring certain implications and challenges which must be met. These are:

(1) the recognition of the mentally handicapped as people with sexual needs and feelings of their own;
(2) the necessity of providing an appropriate form of sexual education geared to their particular needs;
(3) the provision of easily available family planning advice and care. The first two are explored elsewhere in this book, the third is the subject of this chapter.

Establishing a Family Planning Clinic in a Mental Handicap Hospital

By 1972 we had already gone some way towards "normalising" The Manor, a hospital which then cared for about a thousand mentally

241

handicapped residents. We had mixed wards and training departments, patients' clubs, camping and canoeing holidays and fairly free social interactions generally. Our stable, mildly handicapped elderly patients did not wish to alter their ways over much. The hospital had been home to many of them for the greater part of their lives, and they had got their own routine and status in the hospital. Many of them had long-standing ands very stable relatainships with the opposite sex: boy friends and girl friends had grown old together; some now in their sixties and seventies have remained loyal over many years. These long-standing relationships were probably never sexual, but certainly there was mutual affection and support.

It was in relation to the mildly handicapped, turbulent young group that our main anxieties arose. These young people had been admitted to the hospital because of behavioural problems which had brought them into conflict with society in one way or another. They were living in two mixed units, one geared to industrial training, the other to a more domestic type of training. Since that time we have also developed three additional mixed units and a single room 'hostel type' unit whose residents work out in the local community.

In the beginning we felt that with the increasing freedom we had about forty female patients who could be classified as 'high risk' clients. We decided to approach the Family Planning Association for help and advice in setting up a clinic (MacLean 1979). They were most helpful, and a series of meetings took place. We agreed that the clinic would be staffed entirely by FPA trained personnel, and that although occurring within the hospital it should be, and be seen to be, entirely independent of the hospital authorities. If the staff wished to avail themselves of the services of the clinic they would be welcome to do so.

We realised that this clinic would inevitably be unlike an ordinary community clinic because of the nature of the clients, and we have learned as we have gone along. At our first clinic, which was held in very inadequate surroundings, the room being almost a passage way which rapidly became uncomfortably hot, a very hostile, angry and large patient arrived. She stood at the door shouting at us, swearing richly as she questioned my competence in no uncertain terms. She told me I would not know if she was pregnant or not, so what was the point of seeing me? In a way she was right; she proved to have a 'false pregnancy'!

242

Because our patients are often unreliable witnesses, most interviews take much longer than expected. Relevant details have to be extracted from the voluminous case papers, usually to the accompaniment of a non-stop flow of chatter, sometimes hostile but usually friendly. The unco-operative patient also presents a great problem, and much time has to be devoted to examining a difficult girl, with due thought for the influence of any 'sound effects' on waiting patients.

We have learned to be prepared for the unexpected. One girl with primary amenorrhoea, produced vaginal bleeding by persistent self-inflicted trauma so that she would be given a sanitary towel and seem to be "normal". By the time she was first seen in the clinic she had what appeared to be a sinister looking tumour, but which on biopsy showed "simple hypertrophic mucosa indistinguishable from a caruncle". Another used her vagina to carry, on one occasion a razor blade to be used for self-mutilation, and on another her toothbrush. A third woman, mildly handicapped but also schizophrenic, carried her correspondence in her rectum neatly wrapped in a polythene bag. Twice the letters were recovered, but then, unhappily, she felt her safe place had been discovered and she swallowed them instead, which led to serious obstruction requiring laparotomy.

On the whole, the patients seemed to accept the clinic and the clinic staff readily and now, nine years later, visiting the Family Planning Clinic is a normal event. For some of our youngsters the clinic provides a short period during which they have the undivided attention of the doctor or the nurse and in privacy can discuss their fears and anxieties or seek reassurance about their sexual behaviour. We try to personalise the visits as much as possible and much valuable work goes on in the waiting room when the girls are greeted by the Clinic Secretary on arrival. Our main function remains the provision of a contraceptive service but minor gynaecological complaints such as vaginal discharges can be dealt with at the same time.

We are now also providing a menopause clinic facility for a small number of our older ladies. This has proved most rewarding since they are not sophisticated women's magazine readers and are usually referred by observant staff. They give only their own stumbling descriptions of hot flushes and night sweats—"It's all hot, doctor, and comes all over me"; "I can't stay in my bed at night."

Short courses of intermittent hormone replacement therapy have produced encouraging results in the small number dealt with so far.

The clinic still tends to be called the Family Planning Clinic because we are all used to this name and have not succeeded in finding an alternative that has "stuck"—but we are always aware that Birth Control or Minor Gynecological Clinic might be more acceptable—the latter particularly when one remembers that one of our recent "star" patients was a delightful 95 year old with atrophic vaginitis who, when being complimented on her general agility and physical competence offered to show us her telegram from the Queen when it came, "if you're still around"!

Attending the Family Planning Clinic also offers a learning experience for our mildly handicapped girls who, having got used to atttending regularly, are usually quite easily persuaded to accept referral to their local Family Planning Clinic when they finally leave the hospital. In this way we hope to overcome some of the difficulties described by David *et al.* (1976) in their studies of the usage of Family Planning Services provided especially for mentally handicapped clients in the community.

The accurate recording on each woman's Menstrual Chart is considered to be very important—at first as a nursing record, but eventually we always hope they will bring their own cards with them, filled in by themselves, which gives a boost to their confidence and increases their self-repect and sense of responsibility about their contracepton.

The main function of the clinic remains the provision of advice about contraception and the choice of the most appropriate method for each patient.

In deciding on the way in which pregnancy should be avoided, individual needs, personality (including degree of motivation and amount of supervision required) and any medication being taken regularly must all be considered. Mentally handicapped people are as widely varied as any other group and a diversity of solutions to their contraceptive problems is necessary.

Methods Available

We did not consider barrier methods to be appropriate since they depend on motivation and planning ahead, abilities notoriously lacking in our mildly handicapped and impossible for severely mentally handicapped youngsters.

Methods which are appropriate are:

(1) *Hormonal* contraception in the form of (a) the "combined" pill or "progestogen only" pill; or (b) occasionally, Injectables.

(2) *Intra-uterine Devices.*

(3) *Sterilisation.*

Having decided to offer protection then certain criteria must be satisfied. As with all clients, methods offered must be:

convenient — safe — effective

but in addition must require minimal, if any, effort by the mentally handicapped woman to ensure efficiency, since they may well lack the necessary motivation. Nursing or care staff, unless experienced and fully alert to this, may fail to supervice correct taking of the pill and many a youngster will treat it as a game, success being measured by the number of times the staff have been outwitted. This unrealistic approach is a cause of potent concern to clinic staff regarding the possibiity of an unwanted pregnancy, but also as a reflection that the wrong method has been chosen for this particular girl, and also that there has been a failure with the original counselling.

(1) *Hormonal Contraception*

(a) *The 'Pill'.* The 'pill' is now a widely accepted form of contraception and indeed amongst our young population the taking of the pill confers a certain status, the taker being seen as an *active* sexual person or at least capable of being taken as such by the rest of society.

The pill is undoubtedly convenient—how safe is it? There are recognised risks to health and in rare instances to life—and the pill should never be prescribed without proper examination and history taking. The most serious risks of the combined oral contraceptive pill are associated with thromboembolic phenomena and cardiovascular conditions. The risks are all strongly related to age, cigarette smoking, obesity, dose of oestrogen and any predisposing family history or blood pressure, diabetes, etc.

Figures from the longitudinal study of pill users and controls by the Royal College of General Practitioners (Carne *et al.* 1979) showed that the annual mortality risk increases sharply with age. Most of our clinic populations are of course in the younger age bracket—but smoking and obesity are common and very resistant characteristics, and even using the pill as a "desirable" object, attainable by changing habits, has not yet produced dramatic results.

Since oestrogens are thought to be responsible for the serious adverse effects of the combined pill, patients for whom oestrogen is contra-indicated may now be given the "progestogen only" pill. These single hormone pills do seem to be relatively free of side effects—and produce a reasonably reliable level of contraception—comparable with the barrier (condom and cap) methods, and for our young people has the advantage of daily dosage, making it easier to establish a routine.

The combined pill is the most effective contraceptive method—being highly reliable if taken correctly, but may exacerbate pre-existing conditions, which may be found amongst our girls such as depression and diabetes, and especially epilepsy, which presents a particular problem.

Many of our patients are on various types of medication such as anticonvulsant drugs, phenothiaznes, antidepressants, tranquillisers, etc. We try to avoid the use of the oral contraceptive with our epileptic patients particularly, because of the possibility of enzyme induction interfering with the efficiency of the pill, or of possible oestrogen-induced fluid retention adversely affecting epilepsy. But in general we do not favour polypharmacy and this also weighs against the pill if the I.U.D. is acceptable.

(b) *Long-acting Progestogen Injections (Depo-provera).* As the daily "progestogen only" pill has become widely accepted as a reasonably reliable contraceptive without the adverse side-effects attributed to oestrogen, a long-lasting progestogen-only "depot" contraceptive has been developed. This is in the form of an intra-muscular injection of medroxyprogesterone acetate which can be given every 90 days approximately. At present the use of this preparation is still only approved by the Committee on Safety of Medicines for short-term use in the United Kingdom, i.e., when a girl has been immunised against rubella and must NOT get pregnant for at least three months, or when the male partner has undergone vasectomy and the couple are awaiting negative seminal analysis.

246

However it has been used in domiciliary family planning services both in the United Kingdom (Wilson, 1976) and overseas and there is no doubt that for a small number of our mentally handicapped young people this is the method of choice for their contraception. For example, the young mildly handicapped girl who is not motivated to take the pill properly and has had contraceptive failure, pregnancy occurring with an I.U.D. *in situ* or when "on the pill", but who may in the future mature and wish to marry and have children; or the girl of near normal intelligence but with a superimposed psychotic illness who refuses to take the pill or have an I.U.D. but is sexually active and distressed at the thought of pregnancy before being discharged from hospital. For such the injection has been a totally acceptable and efficient method of contraception after the turbulence and failure of previous methods and the trauma of terminations of pregnancy.

In the United States the Federal Drugs Administration has not approved its use as a contraceptive primarily because of fears that it may stimulate cancer of breast or cervix. The evidence for increased risks of cancer of the breast is based on animal studies using beagle bitches, a cancer-prone species of dog, and the relevance of the work to the human female is doubtful. The evidence relating to the cervix is based on slightly increased rates of carcinoma-in-situ found in medroxyprogesterone users in certain series but matched controls were not studied. Other series have failed to show any difference between users and non-users. The F.D.A. concluded that no increased risk could be proved. Similar doubts have been raised in the past about combined oral contraceptives but they continue to be marketed and have F.D.A. approval.

Side effects occurring with medroxyprogesterone acetate are principally in the area of disturbance of menstrual patterns, amenorrhoea being the commonest manifestation. Intermittent or heavy bleeding are much less common disturbances. It is very important that patients should be warned of these possible changes as a sudden cessation of menstruation can be very disturbing psychologically apart from the worry to parents and care staff who may query pregnancy. Menstrual mythology is extensive and often the regular menstruation (except during pregnancy) is seen as an essential method of ridding the body of "bad blood". When this is interrupted great anxiety may be produced as to "where has it gone".

247

Subsequent return of fertility may be delayed following medroxyprogesterone acetate usage and may not return to normal for some months after the last injection, but there is no evidence of any increased risk of fetal abnormalities in pregnancies occurring after discontinuing the treatment.

(2) *Intra-uterine Devices*

I.U.Ds., colloquially known as "the coil", have the great merit of requiring no effort by the user—who may well be oblivious to its presence after the initial fitting.

The other considerable advantage is as protection for the unsettled and impulsive young woman, and we had one such example very early on. A mildly handicapped promiscuous girl absconded one weekend, just six weeks after being fitted with an I.U.D. When she returned some three months later she was thin, neglected and dirty, and there were signs that she had been living rough. She alleged that she had slept around for money and her story was later confirmed by the Social Services Department: she was fortunate to be free from infection and also not pregnant. Adverse effects include expulsion, excessive bleeding and pelvic pain. Expulsion may be complete or partial. Usually, with partial expulsion, the device is easily removed and the patient refitted with particular attention to any underlying cause for the original expulsion. With apparently complete expulsion it becomes necessary to determine whether in fact the threads have been drawn up into the uterus, but the device is still in the correct position—in which case the threads can be drawn down and the patient reassured. If however the device cannot be located, X-rays and ultrasound scans may be used to locate it and if necessary laparoscopic removal from an extra-uterine site may be necessary.

Excessive bleeding and/or pain may occur in up to 10 per cent of users, and if this occurs with our retarded young women, is the cause of much complaint—since motivation, often tenuous to begin with—quickly evaporates if things are not quite right. The abnormal bleeding is usually seen in the early months after fitting and will often settle down spontaneously. There is evidence to suggest that it is connected with increased fibrinolytic activity around the device and the pain with increased prostaglandin synthetase activity.

However, salpingitis, though not common, must not be forgotten in the differential diagnosis.

The problem of ectopic pregnancy must also be considered—since a history of abnormal bleeding and pain may well occur then too, and it is known that there is a higher incidence of tubal pregnancies in I.U.D. users than in females without I.U.Ds. Although an uncommon complication, ectopic pregnancy presents a very real problem since the early diagnosis depends so much on an accurate history and prompt reporting of abnormal bleeding, and yet too intense questioning may alarm our particular clients. We try to incorporate the idea of reporting anything unusual into the taking responsibility for their own menstrual charts eventually.

(3) *Sterilisation*

Sterilisation of mentally handicapped persons remains an emotive subject, posing searching questions for professionals and society alike. The operation of sterilisation is undertaken with the object of preventing further fertility on a permanent basis. At present there are no methods for either sex which can be guaranteed to be reversible—though equally no *absolute* guarantee can be given that the operation will be unequivocally successful.

It is important to stress the exact nature of the operation, what it does, and what it does NOT do, since otherwise families may be expecting the operation to control their relatives' sexual drive or effect some other behavioural change. Some parents have hoped for a return to the "asexual" child again since they have found their offspring's overt sexuality disturbing to themselves. Since neither vasectomy nor tubal division affects sex hormone production, there is usually no change in sex drive at all, only fertility being controlled.

Sterilisation by abdominal hysterectomy may have a place in the treatment of the severely handicapped girl with double incontinence whose family have managed hitherto to care for her at home but feel once menstruation has started that without this operation they may have no alternative to permanent hospital care. For this sort of girl the irrevocable prevention of parenthood is quite incidental.

For whose benefit are retarded people sterilised? Let us consider first mentally handicapped individuals themselves. For some of our young women the experience of pregnancy and certainly of

249

childbirth would be extremely distressing and beyond their comprehension, and may on occasion produce lasting regression. One young woman, first encountered when well into the third trimester of her previously unsuspected pregnancy, had lost what little speech she had and was unable to understand what was happening to her. Following the normal birth of her apparently normal child, she has remained withdrawn and non-communicating and requires considerable support in entering any social situation. She has now been sterilised—but how much better if she had not had to experience first what was for her this appalling shock.

Secondly, a young woman clearly not capable of parenthood and child-rearing, yet able to enjoy heterosexual relationships, may find herself pregnant and being offered termination. This of itself may be devastating to her and if her understanding is such that she can comprehend the implications—how destructive to her self-respect.

Thirdly, sterilization may be requested by an engaged or married mentally handicapped couple who choose for themselves not to become parents, or to limit the size of their families. Some retarded people can and do make realistic decisions based on an appreciation of their limitations (Craft and Craft, 1979) and vasectomy or tubal ligation gives permanent protection.

What about the potential offspring of the mentally handicapped parents, what rights have they? Surely, the right not to be born retarded or born to parents who will not be able to care for them or give them a normal healthy home life in which to develop, no matter how much community support they may have.

The transmission of hereditary defects is put forward as an indication for sterilisation and indeed there would at first sight appear to be substance for this argument. However, the hereditary defects associated with mental handicap are usually seen in the range of severe mental handicap and are often accompanied by physical disabilities as well. These people less likely to be fertile and often are not able to enjoy or engage in heterosexual activity which might lead to pregnancy. The mildly handicapped are usually of the subcultural variety and not affected by the transmissable disorders, but in both cases exceptions will occur and then the most effective method of preventing procreation may well be sterilisation or even, in the severely handicapped girls who are already struggling with menstrual problems—hysterectomy may be indicated.

Parents and care staff may see their responsibilities for the mentally handicapped person, who has been sterilised, as being infinitely easier to bear than when procreation remained a possibility. Parents may fear that they will become responsible for any offspring of their mentally handicapped child. Sterilisation may then be sought allegedly in the interests of the child—whereas the benefit will be more clearly to parent or care staff themselves.

It is perhaps appropriate to mention at this point the case of the 11-year-old girl with Sotos Syndrome whose mother had requested sterilisation for her daughter (*In re D. (a minor)* (1976) 1 All E.R.326.). A consultant paediatrician had agreed, but the child was not sterilised because the case became the subject of a High Court Action and judgement was given that "Sterilisation would deprive the girl of a basic right to bear a child when of age so to do", and the Judge ruled that the operation was neither medically indicated nor necessary and that it would not be in the girl's best interests for it to be performed.

This case raises two further questions: firstly, is it ever necessary or right to sterilise a minor? And secondly, who should give consent when sterilisation of a mentally handicapped person is sought?

The case quoted above produced widespread debate with much involvement of the media, including a televised programme on child sterilisation. Part of the proceedings of that meeting were later published (Focus, 1975). The general conclusion was that to deprive any human being of essential rights without being able to foresee that person's future development could not be in the best interests of the child or of society. It was also felt that the problem was more than a personal problem in the accepted sense and that the full consent of society as well as of parents or guardians would have to be obtained.

The second point concerns the nature of valid and informed consent. There are three elements to consent. First, it must be voluntary, and the decision reached without coercion or the use of bargaining, e.g., "If you have this done you will be able to leave hospital that much sooner". Mentally handicapped people are suggestible and usually anxious to please and seek approval, and it is very easy for them to be subjected to indirect pressures. Secondly, individuals must have all the information made available to them necessary to make a decision, and time taken to explain what is meant. And thirdly, it is of course essential that the person has the mental competence to appreciate what is being consented to and what the implications are. If these three criteria can be met then retarded individuals can give, or withhold, consent on their own account. If this is not so then the consent must be given by others and herein lies the problem. Consent by parent, guardian or the doctor involved could all be held to be possibly suspect, since interests other than those purely related to the mentally handicapped person's well-being might be thought to be present. It would seem that the best solution may well be to extend the D.H.S.S. guide-lines (1975) outlining the informal and formal consultation procedures as in the case of "minors" (under the age of 16) to all those for whom sterilisation is proposed on the grounds of mental handicap.

Thus a multi-professional group, all personally involved with the mentally handicapped person's present welfare, would either meet with the parents or guardians or give advice to them. If this procedure is not satisfactory because of failure to reach a unanimous view, it may be necessary to involve a more formal approach with a local "ethical" committee being involved or a committee being convened by the Secretary of State to consider particular cases.

Sterilisation of mentally handicapped men has received little attention so far. The principal situation in which such a step might be considered is where a mildly handicapped but promiscuous man presents a risk to vulnerable girls in an institution or in a local community. Sterilisation, though controlling fertility, would not offer any protection against rape (which may be the greater problem presented by these men); it is also likely to be irreversible thereby depriving the handicapped man of any future possibility of fathering a child, should his behavioural problems come under control. An alternative to sterilisation is drug control of his sexual behaviour. This would certainly offer greater protection to society, diminishing the risk of rape as well as pregnancy. Against this there may be some personality change or physical side-effects and the administration and taking of the drugs themselves need continuous supervision which, like the oral contraceptive with the females, may present difficulty to nursing and care staff. However, drug therapy is reversible and if the man is able to give informed consent these facts must be discussed with him: if he is not able to give his own consent, the facts must be weighed by the multi-professional group advising his relatives or guardians.

Conclusion

As we continue to move slowly towards our goal of full integration for the mentally handicapped into their own local communities it is approriate that we should consider afresh the sexuality of this most deprived section of our society. A constructive approach to their psycho-sexual needs by way of education and counselling in the use of contraceptive techniques will not only help in personal adjustment but will make possible one more step in the direction of normality and ultimate integration.

REFERENCES

Carne, S., Chamberlain, G. and MacEwen, J. (1979). *Handbook of Contraceptive Practice* (revised 1978). Prepared for the Standing Medical Advisory Committee of Central Health Services Council by representatives of the Royal College of Obstetricians and Gynecologists and the Royal College of General Practitioners. London: DHSS; Scottish Home and Health Department; Welsh Office.

Craft, A. and Craft, M. (1979). *Handicapped Married Couples*. London: Routledge and Kegan Paul.

David, H.P., Smith, J.D. and Friedman, E. (1976). Family Planning Services for Persons Handicapped by Mental Retardation. *Amer.J.Public Health 66*, 11, 1053–7.

Department of Health and Social Security (1975). *Sterilization of Children under Sixteen Years of Age: Discussion paper*. London: DHSS.

Focus (1975). Current Attitudes in Medical Ethics: Child Sterilisation. *J.Med.Ethics* 1, 163–7.

MacLean, R. (1979). Sexual Problems and Family Planning Needs with the Mentally Handicapped in Residential Care. *Brit.J.FamilyPlanning 4*, 4, 13–15.

Wilson, E. (1976). Use of Long-Acting Depot Progestogen in Domiciliary Family Planning. *Brit.Med.J.* 2, 1435–7.

CHAPTER 12

Sexuality Counselling with Developmentally Disabled Couples

Linda Andron

Counselling couples around issues of marriage, parenthood and sexuality can be an extremely rewarding and challenging experience. In this chapter, I will share the knowledge gained from the many couples I have counselled over the last ten years.

Who Were the Couples and Where Did They Come From?

Over the years, many labels have been applied to the population at hand: idiot, imbecile, mentally retarded, and most recently, mentally handicapped and developmentally disabled. I believe it is the latter which most appropriately characterizes the group with which I have worked. All of them were labelled mentally retarded as children and virtually all were educated in special classes. Their tested IQs as children ranged from 50-85. When the definition of mental retardation shifted from one to two standard deviations below the mean, most of this group were no longer considered retarded. What were they then? I believe that these couples are best described as developmentally disabled within the broadest definition of this term, now the policy of the United States government.[1]

Most would probably be diagnosed specifically as learning disabled, had they been born 20 years later. Many have some type of demonstrable brain damage, evidenced by speech or mild motor impediments or seizure disorder. Several of them would fit the category of mild mental retardation, some with additional demonstrable neurological or specific learning deficits. I have not had extensive experience with the moderately or trainable mentally retarded. Colleagues have recently met two such couples and hope to learn much from them. While many have developed emotional symptomatology, a diagnosis of personality disorder can be made in only two cases. This is in sharp contrast to the experience described by the Crafts.[2]

In contrast to the experiences of the Crafts (1979) and Janet Mattinson (1975), histories of deprivation are rare in our population. The two women diagnosed as personality disordered are the only ones who share such a history. Most of these couples came from middle to upper middle class families, with a few having well-known parents in the television and movie community. The rest come from lower middle class homes with some history of family instability, but in which their basic needs were always met. Most of the couples grew up in families where their limitations were in sharp distinction to the abilities both of their parents and siblings. Almost all grew up at home, with only a few attending boarding school.

The population varies greatly with regard to age, length of marriage, living arrangements and treatment(s) employed. Ages ranged from 20-50, and length of marriage varied from pre-marital involvement to 22 years, with many having been married as long as 10-15 years. Nearly all the couples resided independently in the community, including two graduates and one active couple from an independent living training programme. Two lived in board-and-care settings. There were four divorces or annulments. Eleven couples were seen in group therapy, two in conjoint premarital counselling, three in conjoint marital therapy, and four in intensive sexual dysfunction therapy. Three couples were involved in discussions leading to the production of a videotape.[3] (See Figure 1 for detailed description.)

How did I come to know these couples? An initial interest in the needs of married couples emerged as a result of meeting a few disabled couples via both regular community contacts and a county social services department. Sensing the companionship that marriage afforded them while simultaneously recognizing that most of them felt strong isolation from all but family, I formed a group to provide both socialization and counselling. Referrals from other interested professionals soon followed, as the the benefits of this kind of group experience (as well as other forms of counselling offered to group members) became more and more apparent. Clients have also referred themselves for the group and marital or pre-marital and more recently sexual counselling. The two women (Nancy and Betty) with diagnoses of personality disorder and histories of deprivation referred themselves at the suggestions of agencies for issues related to child development and care.

255

	IQ Range	Living Arrangement	Length of Marriage (years)	Marital Status	Sterilization	Type of Therapy	Sexual Difficulty	Children
Ruth and Jim	R: 60's / J: 80's	Own apt.	4	Married	Vasec.	G	E, I, M, O, RE	None
Judy and Bill	J: 60's / B: 80's	Own apt.	22	Married	Hyster. Vasec.	G, I, M, VT	E, I, O, P, RE	None
Kay and Jeremy	K: 80's / J: 70's	Own apt.	1½	Married	None	G, S	I, O, P, PE, SA	None
Carrie and Will	C: 60's / W: Av.	Parent's home	8	Married	Vasec.	G	I, M, O	
Caroline and Ronald	C: Low / R: Av.	Own apt.	11	Married	None	G, I, M, S Genetic	D, I, O, P, RE	One
Susan and Norman	S: 70's / N: Low Av.	Own apt.	8	Married	None	S, just beginning	E, I, O, P, PE	None
Gina and Alan	G: Low Av. / A: Low	Own apt.	13	Married	Vasec.	G, M	E, I, O,	One
Robin and John	R: Low Av. / J: Low Av.	Own apt.	12	Married	None	G, I VT and Genetic	I, O, PE	One
Sharon and Robert	S: 50's / R: 80's	Board and Care	6	Married	None	G, Genetic	Unknown	One
June and Donald	J: 70's / D: 50's	Independent living project		Married	Vasec.	G, PM	E, I, O, P Pain on i'course(male), SA	One
Nina and Ned	N: 60's / N: 80's	Parents and own apt.		Engaged / Engaged, never married	None	G, VT	Unknown	None
Paula and Richard	60's	Board and Care	8/12	Divorced	None	G, S	I, O, P, SA	None
Rachel and	R: 80's				Tubal	I, PM.		None

					Vasc. Tubal Ligation	G, M, S	I, O, RE	
Jim and Mark	J: 80's M: 80's	Own apt.	1½	Divorced		I, PT	O	None
Nancy	Av.	Own apt.	3	Divorced				Three
Betty and Carl	B: 70's C: Av.	Her mother's apt. mission, motel	3	Deceased	None	I	Unknown	Two

CODE

Type of therapeutic involvement

G = group
I = individual
M = marital
PM = pre-marital
PT = parent training
S = sexual counselling or therapy
VT = involved in production of video-tape

Type of Sexual Problem

D = dyspareunia (pain on intercourse)
E = erectile dysfunction
I = issues of initiation, frequency, communication or technique
M = medical aspects (seizures, muscular weakness)
O = orgasmic dysfunction
P = phobic avoidance or specific phobias
PE = premature or rapid ejaculation
RE = retarded ejaculation
SA = sexual assault (past history of rape or other sexual assault)

Figure 1: Details of couples counselled

Many common issues have arisen with all of the couples with whom I have worked. The most salient in my experience have centred around issues of relations with families, communication between partners, housing, procreation, sterilization and sexual dysfunction. Our experience has also shown some common threads in the life history of these couples, which seem to underlie the development of these concerns. From all of the above plus our experience in dealing with these, I have found significant implications for practice. Let us begin then with a discussion of the various issues raised in counselling developmentally disabled couples.

Relations with Families

A common issue raised by many couples is that of the response of families to their marriage. Many experienced severe opposition, the nature of which has taken many forms. In several cases, the opposition has been to the concept of marriage itself, with the parents feeling that their child could not handle the resonsibility. For example, Paula and Richard married against the wishes of both of their families. Richard's father based his opposition on the fact that Richard could not support Paula. It had not occurred to him that the same Social Security payments which had supported each of them individually would do the same for them as a couple. In other cases, the opposition was to the particular person chosen.

Families do not always oppose the marriage. In fact, there were two cases in which the families arranged the marriage. One broke up after only a year and one-half. The other has lasted 22 years in spite of ongoing strife. Bill describes his family's arrangement of his marriage as follows:

> See, our family got us together and said we had to get married. . . . So, I mean, you know, I mean, I didn't have any decision to make on it, you know. They said we were going to get married and, you know. . . . I told my family I'd like to have some responsibility and, you know, and I thought it might be nice if I got married and, you know. . . .[3]

One concern often raised by families is what will happen if the marriage fails. An example of this was Ned's family's reaction when he told them of his engagement to Nina:

> You've been hurt by her so many times before. You know the divorce rate in California and all that. It was a big thing; I felt like it was three against one.[3]

Many of the couples married in spite of strongly voiced family concerns and opposition. In some cases, the marriages were strengthened by the couple's determination to prove themselve.

What of family relations after marriage? Most of the couples complained of over-involvement on the part of their families. In some cases, such as Ruth and Jim's, both partners felt the same way about their families' attempts to intervene in their lives.

> Ruth's sister has retained ongoing opposition to her marriage and has repeatedly threatened her with institutional placement. Resisting this pressure and winning the battle against her in regard to Social Security payeeship has been a major uniting force in their marriage.

On the other hand, issues of family involvement were an ongoing source of conflict for others. For some, this has been a negative factor, but has not necessarily undermined the marriage. This was the case for Judy and Bill. They had ongoing arguments about how much to depend on their families and whose family was right in a given situation. While Bill functions very competently as a supervising custodian, at home he is content to allow the family to make all his decisions—including the purchase of his clothes. While Judy voices her dissatisfaction, she does not assert herself in opposing family decisions. During a home visit for the purpose of videotaping, they shared the following feelings with us:

> J—I resent you always going to your family.
> B—I mean, my mother has more experience than you.
> J—Well, try me.

In response to the question, "Do you ever want to tell your parents that you can do things on your own?" Bill replied:

> No, I don't think so, because I don't have the qualifications for doing things on my own.

Judy on the other hand, replied:

> Some things I like to go to them for, and other things I call and say, "Ya, I want help." And other times I say, "Why don't you let me make my own decisions. You can't live my life for me. If I need help, I'll come to you, but otherwise leave me alone."

Where one partner shows great dependence on parents, often to the exclusion of the partner, serious problems ensue. For Paula and Richard it was one of the issues which ended their brief marriage. Richard was not able to accept being left at the board-and-care home, while Paula went home to spend frequent weekends with her mother. Kay and Jeremy reached a compromise on this same issue, and Kay has come to accept Jeremy's visits home and learn to value her solitary leisure. In their case, there is conflict over what Kay feels is Jeremy's preference for his mother and his unwillingness to stand up for Kay in a disagreement. Kay, on 'the other hand, espouses great anger toward her own mother and expresses a burning desire to be independent of her, but is unable to detach herself in reality. She has volunteered at the school which employs her mother and recently moved within close proximity. There appears to be a common denominator in these two situations. Both Richard and Kay felt rejected since placement in boarding school in their late latency years, and view adult acceptance by their mothers as the most valued reinforcement.

There has also been a common denominator in the families I have met. While their level of involvement has been highly problematic for many couples, their sincere concern and interest in the couples' well-being has been obvious. It seems that the negative prognoses and protect-and-shelter advice received by families when their children were diagnosed 15-20 years ago have had a major effect which does not shift automatically because of newly developing philosophies.

Communication

Communication difficulties between partners is a common theme raised both before and after marriage both by the couples and their families. Many parents express serious concern about their children's abilities to handle this aspect of a marital relationship. Just how much alike or different were the communication problems of our couples to the "average" couple? When we asked Judy and Bill if they felt their marriage was different from that of non-handicapped couples, they both said no. However, Bill went on to add:

Except that some marriages, I mean, they are more normal. There are a lot of couples that aren't handicapped, mentally retarded, that means a little slow. And they are able to cope with things maybe better than we are in a lot of ways.

Picture Judy interrupting with her own strong feelings about communication:

They can communicate better than we can. They can talk things over the way we should learn to do. It (marriage) could be wonderful if we'd learn to talk things over, you know. Like when he greets me when he comes home. I know he's tired when he comes home. The family is always throwing it up to me. But, I'm lonesome. Like most husbands, instead of going right to the refrigerator, they whistle "Honey, I'm home," and that gives the wife a wonderful feeling and she comes running. Him, I never know. He just ignores me and treats me like a piece of the furniture.[3]

Housing

Another common concern relating to marriage was around the question of housing. Those couples who were able to manage in their own apartments faced the problem of being able to afford increasingly high rents. For others, who felt they needed or wanted a more sheltered setting, other problems arose. In board-and-care facilities, privacy and the shared functions of married life become central difficulties. Such was the case for Paula and Richard. When they married, they were given one bedroom in a two bedroom unit shared with another couple. Beyond sharing a room and having conjugal relations, they did not function as a couple. They continued to receive their weekly allowances separately and did their laundry separately according to previously established schedules. Their room was cleaned by a maid and they ate their meals in the common dining hall. Their sexual relations were complicated by the fact that they never knew when the other couple would walk in on them.

For Sharon and Robert, the second couple living in a board-and-care facility, the issue was finding a setting that could accommodate both themselves and their expected child. This experience is best described in their own words:

> Family care is where the caretaker would take care of the baby and treat us like kids. We don't like that. We are adults. We are married and are expecting a child. We're like everyone else. We have problems. But we have an additional problem—we're handicapped. And her handicap [only a stub on one arm and mild to moderate retardation] is more serious than mine [cerebral palsy and borderline intellectual functioning] and I understand that. And we're really going to try to overcome it. There are all kinds of obstacles ahead of us, but we'll take them as they come.[3]

This particular story, unfortunately, had a tragic ending. Unable to find the appropriate sheltered setting, they attempted to live in their own apartment in spite of their total lack of preparation. In the end, they felt forced to place their child in foster care.

261

Procreation

The question of whether or not a developmentally disabled couple should have children comes up often in practice. More often than not, however, I have found that the decision has been made prior to the couple entering counselling, and that it is the sequela of this decision that we face. In the case of those who have decided against child-rearing, two salient points stand out. The first is that most of the couples we counselled have retained the idea that adoption is a viable alternative for them. The second is their desire not to bring a handicapped child into the world. Often, after sterilization they discover that they have been misinformed about one or both issues. Such was the experience of Will and Carrie. Both Will's seizure disorder and Carrie's speech defect and mild mental retardation have been related to birth trauma. In spite of this, they were told that their children would be handicapped, since all handicapped people bear handicapped children. On this basis, they agreed to sterilization. When they joined our couples group and found two of the couples parenting normal children, they became extremely angry at being misled.

It has been the rare situation in our group's experience that parents, doctors, or other concerned individuals have been honest about their reasons for advising against child-rearing. "You wouldn't want to bring a handicapped child into the world" appears to be easier to say than "I don't feel you have the capacity to raise a child." The second question is totally begged by those who advised these couples that they could always adopt a child.

An issue often brought up by couples and their families relates to the relative intelligence of the children-to-be. What will happen if the children are smarter than their parents? Ned and Nina's response was:

> It wouldn't bother me. I know there are lots of people in this world who are smarter than me. It wouldn't bother me. Matter of fact, I WOULD BE GLAD. Maybe this kid could go to law school or be a doctor at UCLA. . . . If the children were way smarter than us then maybe they could teach us a few things.
> L.A.: Do you think it would hurt the children if they were smarter?
> I don't think so. I think it would make them very proud.

Those who do have children have expressed some concern about this point.

262

Another theme commonly raised is the need for and value of genetic counselling and how to interpret its results. Three of the couples sought genetic counselling on their own. Two, reassured that their risk factor appeared no higher than for a "normal" couple, have since had children. In the third case, a higher risk factor based on family history was established, and the issue of how this was interpreted arose. Rachel showed some structural deformities in the neck and shoulder. Since her half-sister also presented with deformities of the jaw bone, she was informed that her risk for congenital abnormality in her offspring might be slightly higher than average, approximately 10 per cent. This figure was repeated over and over by her mother-in-law to the point that Rachel lost the context and came to believe that she had only a 10 per cent chance of having a normal child. On this basis, she agreed to be sterilized. Her mother-in-law later said that she had really been concerned about her ability to raise children, but did not want to say so and therefore pushed the genetic aspect.

There are no clear answers to the question of whether or not developmentally disabled couples can raise children. Literature in this area is scant. No long-term studies taking into account all the relevant variables have yet been completed. In my experience, parents who experience difficulties in childrearing share histories of neglect and abuse themselves. Thus, any conclusions regarding their ability to parent are compounded by difficulties in elucidating the factors of intellectual deficit and abuse and neglect as children. At the same time, only those having difficulties are known to our agency or other parts of the service delivery system. We cannot know what percentage of those labelled developmentally disabled have gone on to parent and have blended into the community at large.

What are the sequels for those who decide against childbearing? All of the couples I have counselled who have reached this conclusion bear feelings of sadness over the decision. Many express regret that they yielded to the pressure of others. Anger is expressed toward those who were less than honest and who fostered fantasies of adopted children. Those who based their decision on their own determination of their limitations, express feelings of distress at what they see as one more failure in their ability to do what normal people do. This has been underscored in the work of others (Sabagh and Edgerton 1962; Andron and Sturm 1973).

Sterilization

The decision to seek sterilization would seem to be predicated on a prior decision to terminate one's ability to procreate. . . . It does not always follow, however, that these couples or individual partners have first gone through the process of deciding against having children before seeeking sterilization. For many, it was the price they had to pay for the family's support of their marriage or move to independent living. For several, the issue of children was left open with promises of surgical reversal or adoption. Most of the couples I have counselled were confronted with the issues relative to sterilization prior to being referred for counselling. For several, there was no counselling other than that provided by the families. Many later realized that they had not fully understood the reasons for or finality of such a move, or even its relation to their ability to procreate.

A predominant issue raised is the question of determining the person's fertility prior to sterilization. In Jim's case, a careful medical assessment and fertility determination would have revealed that he had a genetic disorder that rendered him sterile. This would have avoided the severe pain he felt in yielding to family pressure and having the vasectomy that so violated his religious beliefs.

For Mark, a prior attempt to determine fertility would have led to the discovery of a serious problem in sexual functioning (retarded ejaculation). A series of severe difficulties which eventually led to the breakup of the marriage might have been avoided.

Mark's parents arranged a marriage for him with a girl from New York. Generally compliant to their wishes, he readily agreed to the marriage and a vasectomy. Following the surgery, for which no prior test of fertility was made, a semen specimen was needed by the doctor to determine the surgery's effectiveness. Mark was unable to produce the ejaculate. He was assured it would be all right after the marriage. Following the wedding, there were daily calls from the family to see if the marriage had been consummated and the specimen taken to the doctor. The couple did not undertsand the different procedures required to obtain these two goals. Much pressure was put on the wife. After a period of sexuality education did not suffice, Mark and Jill were referred to a colleague for sex therapy. He was diagnosed as having primary retarded ejaculation and after extensive therapy, including the use of a surrogate, he was able to produce the specimen and consummate the marriage. However, by this time the fabric of the marriage had been so torn that divorce ensued.

264

A related question is whether or not a couple is in fact sexually active. After agreeing to sterilization on the basis of genetic counselling, Rachel (discussed above) questioned why this was so urgent since she and her husband never had successful penetration.

The most pressing issue with regard to sterilization concerns the questions of what is informed consent and what constitutes a "voluntary sterilization". Current regulations of the United States Department of Health and Human Services prohibit persons under 21, people living in institutions, or who are adjudicated to be mentally incompetent from being sterilized at their own or another's consent.[4] Most of the couples I have counselled do not fit any of these categories and so are presumed capable of giving their own informed consent. In my experience, it is these people who supposedly can provide informed consent and thus be voluntarily sterilized who often end up with an "involuntary" sterilization from which their more handicapped peers are protected by virtue of current regulations. Because of their limited knowledge, their desire to please, and their pattern of yielding to authority figures, they have a tendency to give in to pressure. And because of their general suggestibility, they are unable to test the validity of the information they are given regarding the risks of having a handicapped child, the permanence of the procedure, or the possibility of adoption. Such was the case for Nina.

> When she was reportedly told by her father and gynecologist that she was missing a chromosome and would, therefore, have handicapped children, she agreed to a sterilization. When she told various professionals she was dealing with of this, she was advised that only genetic counselling, not gynecologic examination could tell her about her chromosomes and their effect on future offspring. She decided to postpone the surgery. When she did so, the father threatened suit against all the professionals involved, told her that he would block her move to independent living and cut off all her access to advice and counsel other than his own. She subsequently followed through on the surgery and several months later attempted to take her own life.

A major issue around sterilization has to do with its effect on sexual functioning. Among my cases most of the men who had vasectomies reported erectile problems, either beginning or getting worse following surgery. Though all of the sterilizations were technically voluntary, most were signed under family pressure. It may, therefore, be that in consenting, these people have relinquished some aspects of autonomy and the surgery represents an assault on their identity as men.

It has been noted that in some men concerns about the sexual effects of a vasectomy may cause difficulty on a psychogenic basis. men who equate masculinity with the ability to reproduce may have difficulties. Problems have also been noted in men with hypochondriasis, concerns about their masculinity and pre-existing sexual difficulties (Ziegler 1970; Kolodny *et al* 1979).

Sexual Dysfunction

I have been involved in work with developmentally disabled couples for the last ten years. Problems relating to family, communication, housing, procreation and sterilization have been pre-eminent through all these years. It has, however, only been in the last three to four years that couples have raised issues of sexual functioning. Until 1979, the subject only came up during counselling when questions were asked. It is only since 1980 that I have personally seen couples referring themselves with the specific complaint of sexul dysfunction. It seems that interest in sexual dysfunction which was focussed on "normal" couples in the 1960s by the work of Masters and Johnson, and the subsequent interest in the sexual needs of the physically handicapped that filled the 1970s may now focus on the learning handicapped in the 1980s.

As part of the overall therapy in my couples group, the clients requested some focus on issues of sexuality. Before beginning this, both the level of knowledge and sexual practices and difficulties were individually assessed. It was at this time that I discovered that all members of the group presented with some level of sexual difficulty. Only two couples had made prior mention of difficulty, and only one had ever sought therapy.

For a detailed individual analysis of the difficulties presented, the reader is referred back to Figure 1. All of the women reported some orgastic difficulties. Many also reported problems with arousal and lubrication. However, language barriers and the non-objective criteria for measuring this made it hard to assess. Erectile dysfunction was the most common complaint among the men, with many reporting retarded or total lack of ejaculatory capacity even when erections were obtained. Three other men reported premature or rapid ejaculation. Several women presented with pain on intercourse. Only Caroline was diagnosed as having dyspareunia, as the others described their "pain" as being associated with the discomfort of the husband lying on top of them in the missionary position (the only one they knew and used). One male reported pain on intercourse. This proved to be due to improper cleansing of the foreskin. Phobias and phobic avoidance of sexual contact or specific practices was reported by more than half the couples. Issues of communication, frequency, and basic lack of knowledge regarding sexual response and effective stimulation techniques were presented by all couples. In addition, aspects of the effects of medical problems (such as seizure or muscle weakness and spasm) created difficulties for two.

Two of the women presented with problems related to past sexual assaults. In both cases, there was some level of complicity on their part with basic exploitation of their rights. The women reported that these experiences had faded and did not affect their pre-marital sex. Both became phobic about being touched following their marriages.

In our experience and that of colleagues, the overall issues presented by disabled couples more closely approximate those of normal couples than they do those of the physically handicapped with whom this group is often linked. The main factor in this is that their problems appear to have a learned and emotional, rather than a physiological basis. Those who are physically disabled from birth, as opposed to those disabled in adolescence or adulthood, share some common concern regarding self-image and feelings of not being as sexual as the "normal" population.

The list of learned causes of sexual dysfunction described by Kaplan (1974) fit both the average and developmentally disabled couple. The first of these is sexual ignorance. Most of our group did not know that there was a difference between the clitoris and the vagina. Two reported not knowing that one must thrust after intromission. Several had no idea that women had orgasms, and others believed that women ejaculated on orgasm. Many of these same things have been reported by "normal" couples, but both the quality and quantity of these in the belief systems of the couples with which I have worked have made them appear to represent caricatures of the "normal".

Fear of failure and the anxiety brought on by the demand for performance are points raised by many who seek sex therapy, and were almost uniformly reported by the couples I have seen. This is exacerbated by the excessive need to please a partner, often for fear that he or she will leave otherwise.

Failure to communicate is probably the central issue expressed by these couples. For most, communication skills were not fostered during childhood. They report being talked to or around, rather than being talked with.

The cultural norms and constrictive upbringing that can lead to adult sexual functional problems are enforced even more strictly for those labelled deviant. Most of the couples we see express severe guilt and anxiety about sexuality. They report extremely negative feelings about expressing any part of their sexuality that does not fit the culturally normative expectation of precreation.

Several common themes have arisen among the couples seen in intensive therapy and those involved in the general sexuality awareness that is part of our group counselling. By far the most common point raised among the women was the lack of understanding of what was meant by orgasm. Others included not knowing of the existence of the clitoris or its function in female orgasm, and believing that simultaneous orgasm was essential (to the point that one woman felt that lack of this was why her children had been born retarded).

Many of the men did not see alternatives to rapid ejaculation, and yet somehow knew that it was a problem. If intercourse is seen as being only for the purpose of procreation, then rapid ejaculation is a plus rather than a minus. It is only when sexuality takes on the dimension of pleasure that lasting longer is valued. A humorous note to be added is that in this case it is not a failure to be slow. Other issues raised by the men included not knowing that some loss of erection or problems in obtaining one on a transient basis is normal, or that difficulties in achieving ejaculation required attention.

The women raised issues regarding their partners which centered around desiring more touching as well as paying attention to their own needs. However, few were aware of exactly what they needed in the way of stimulation to achieve satisfaction. It was most often the wives who reported that they had to initiate sexual contacts, and it was also the women who expressed a desire for more sexual activity than they were currently having.

Both men and women expressed discomfort with self-pleasuring and many with being naked. All held strong beliefs that sexual contact was dangerous during menstruation. A few of the men had no concept of what menstruation was and thought their wives were bleeding. All of the couples have indicated a need to expand the range of positions they used in intercourse.

The most uniform need for help presented has been in the area of communication. The most common problem area is that of initiation. Communicating within the session regarding pleasurable as well as negative feelings and specific requests for stimulation was also raised. An interesting point raised by two couples was that of their desire for an asexual marriage.

In addition to the couples counselled within the group context, I have now seen four couples in intensive sexual dysfunction therapy. These couples have shared in common not the severity, but the multiplicity of their symptoms. Thus, Caroline and Ronald presented with dyspareunia (pain on intercourse), phobic responses, orgasmic dysfunction, retarded ejaculation, and issues of initiation and frequency. Kay and Jeremy presented with premature ejaculation, secondary orgasmic dysfunction, phobias around nudity, being touched, being interrupted, difficulties of initiation and a desire to learn other positions. Susan and Norman presented with premature ejaculation, erectile dysfunction associated with diabetic neuropathy, and phobic avoidance of sex on Susan's part. Paula and Richard presented with phobic avoidance, rapid ejaculation and orgasmic dysfunction as well as severe marital problems which eventually led to an annulment.

For all the couples requiring intensive therapy, sexual problems were intertwined with marital problems. It should be noted that this occurs throughout the "normal" population as well; however, some people experience severe sexual difficulties within the context of a good relationship.

Only Paula and Richard's marriage was severely in jeopardy. It appears that once married, Paula regretted her action and began to find intimacy itself punishing. Past "rapes" were suddenly resurrected and a phobic avoidance of sexuality developed. When the issue of the rapes was raised, the anger at Richard surfaced and ultimately led to the annulment. Premarital sex had apparently been relatively rewarding in spite of rapid ejaculation.

Susan also reported enjoyable premarital sex and dates her phobic avoidance of love-making to one occasion early in marriage

269

when Norman struck her after she dropped some eggs.

Kay and Jeremy's marriage is characterized by his basic dependence on her to initiate in all areas of their lives, her inability to accept positives, her striking ability to deal out negatives, plus his constant worrying about chores and other responsibilities. The question of family relationships was also pressing. All of this was reflected in their problems in sexual functioning.

Caroline believed that her sexual problems came first and led to her marital problems. She related pain upon intercourse to their first faltering attempts. Seeking help from her mother-in-law, she was told that if her husband did not ejaculate, he would go crazy. Fearing the pain, she began to distance herself from Ronald. Finally, they went for sexual counselling through the family practice unit of a university hospital, where they were told they could not be helped and should instead seek marital therapy. By the time they referred themselves to us for sex therapy, the marital conflicts had become severe.

Development of the Psycho-social Script

We believe there are common elements in the life histories of these couples and in most developmentally disabled couples which may account for many of the difficulties arising in marriage which we have discussed.

These are best understood within the context of John Gagnon's view of sexuality as "social learning development perspective" (Gagnon, 1977). According to this model, sexuality is not a congenital force or instinct, but an awareness we acquire in the process of development. Behaviour and attitudes develop as we interact with others and receive their messages about what is right and wrong.

> The idea of a script, a device for guiding action and for understanding it, is a metaphor drawn from the theatre. Viewing conduct as scripted is a way of organizing our thinking about behavior. Scripts are the plans that people may have in their heads for what they are doing and what they are going to do, as well as being devices for remembering what they have done in the past. Scripts justify actions which are in accord with them and cause us to question those which are not—A script is simpler than the activity we perform, often more limited and schematic. It's like a blueprint or a road map or recipe, giving directions, but not specifying

270

everything that must be done (Gagnon 1977).

For many adults raised in average homes, the messages regarding the who, what, when, where, and why read something like this: We are to grow up and marry someone of similar age, race, ethnicity, religion, and social class. Then and only then are we to have sex, which is defined as intercourse, for the purpose of procreation. We are to have intercourse in private, usually in our bedroom, and most often under the cover of darkness.

The basic script is reinforced by what we see in magazines and on television. However, from reading books, peer contacts, and life experience, we expand our script somewhat to include a broader definition of the who, what, when, where, and why.

The situation is a little different for most developmentally disabled and mentally handicapped individuals. First, they do not have access to the other sources of information that affect the broader population. As Ellen, a graduate of classes for the educable mentally retarded tells us:

> They need it (sex education) more because they don't talk about it like, let's say, at lunch time or during breaks in school than regular kids do, and so regular kids get information from here and there. Maybe it is wrong information. It usually is wrong, but still they need to . . .

In spite of this, they often manage to pick up a great deal of street knowledge. However, like the Crafts, we have found that this is usually without much understanding of what the words convey or of the facts of sexuality (Craft and Craft 1978).

The couples I have treated seem to have gained a great deal of information from television. This has led to their extensive knowledge about babies born in six months or eleven months, ectopic pregnancy, twins with two different fathers, but not the more common ways these things occur. Television watching has also reinforced the concept that normalcy means marriage and children.

For the mentally handicapped/developmentally disabled, doing what is seen as normal has become the central focus of the script they live as adults. Thus, the mentally handicapped/developmentally disabled person grows up with the sexual script of sexuality = intercouse = procreation = normalcy. While receiving these messages, he or she is almost always being told that he/she will not be able to parent; or in some cases, even to marry.

Other factors have played a role in making decisions regarding sterilization, parenting, and sexual functioning. For many, the

271

question of *who* has been particularly painful. Robert, explaining why he chose to marry Sharon, said of his father's reaction:

> He wanted me to pick a woman who was almost normal. And I told him, "Dad, I've tried, but almost all the girls who were normal said 'Hey, I don't want you'."[3]

The *where* and *when* has also been a point of confusion for many. I have found that in general a higher standard of behaviour has been imposed on those labelled as disabled than on the general population. One might say that when the package is damaged we inspect the contents more closely. It is as though when people know something is wrong they tend to watch more vigilantly for inappropriate behaviour.

The message that sexuality is for marriage and in private becomes more conflicting when privacy is not respected and the family or others may literally walk into the home, even after marriage. This happened to Judy and Bill. Judy's uncle (married to her mother) had the key to her house. One day while making love, which Bill told us he already believed to be dirty, Judy's uncle walked in on them. This led to an almost total curtailment of sexual activity for the remainder of their 22 years of marriage. As was the case with Richard and Paula, where do sexual relations occur in a shared apartment with no lock on the bedroom door?

To the *what* question have come complicating messages, for example masturbation causing the very thing they struggle against—mental handicap (not to mention "warts and hair on the hands").

Thus, a very constricted script develops with a clear message that to be normal one must marry and have children. Sexuality as an expression of relationship, sensuality as a dimension of pleasure, touching as a means of communication, have been absent in the scripts of the couples with whom I have worked.

Practice Notes

What does all this mean for the clinician's involvement with developmentally disabled couples? And what implications are there for those working with younger children and their families and providing sex education and counselling to the adolescents and young adults who may become couples in the future?

The PLISSIT Model

This can easily be examined within the framework of the PLISSIT model developed by Jack Annon (Annon, 1974). This model was created to provide four levels of approach to the brief treatment of sexual problems within a learning theory framework. I believe that this model has much wider applicability and can help in ordering the sexuality education, counselling, and therapy for developmentally disabled individuals and couples. The four levels are (1) Permission, (2) Limited Information, (3) Specific Suggestions and (4) Intensive Therapy (See Figure 2).

In Annon's model, the first level, permission-giving applies to allowing clients to engage in behaviours in which they are already engaging, but which they believe are abnormal; or permission to engage in behaviours they have been avoiding. For developmentally disabled, permission-giving has implications on many levels. Both those involved in early diagnostic counselling and those working with adults can readily employ this approach. For instance, when asked for long-term prognostic evaluations of the

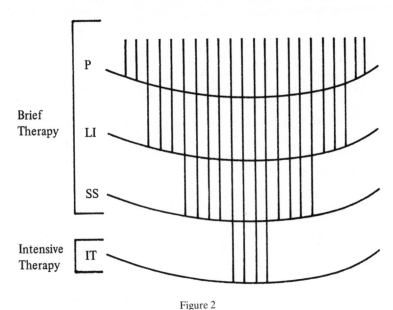

Figure 2

The PLISSIT Model (Annon 1974)

child's functioning, the clinician can use a permission-giving approach to help the family hope and plan for the child's maximum independent functioning and sexual development.

Clinicians must also use this approach to give developmentally disabled individuals permission to follow a life-course which may or may not include marriage, but is still seen as normal. The same applies to children. This is a vital message to give as early in counselling as possible. The parent or other caretaker plays the most significant role in shaping the sexual script. The challenge for them is to give the young person permission to see marriage as possible and at the same time to see being unmarried as both possible and normal. Here, the clinician will need to move to the levels of providing information about what is known on the subject of marriage and mental handicap and specific suggestions as to what parents can do to facilitate development of the most positive script possible. For instance, one might suggest that they bring to their children's attention friends and acquaintances who are unmarried and yet enjoying their lives. The clinician will need to empathize with the very difficult task the parent faces in trying to do this.

I have gained much valuable information from knowing these couples in depth. One piece of information I have come to find vital to share with families of adolescents and young adults regards the slower pace of development of this population and its effect on marriage and sexuality. Most of the couples I have helped married in their late 20's and 30's and have reported that adolescent issues lingered well into their 20's.

A few of the couples married when one or both partners were quite young. Three of these marriages broke up. Betty is an excellent example of a woman who married before she had resolved many remaining adolescent conflicts.

Betty married at age 19 and experienced a great deal of conflict during her three years of marriage. . . . Following the birth of her two daughters, her husband (in his 30's) died of a heart atttack. She then found herself experiencing the adolescent rebellion and desire to explore what she had previously been unable to express. Her home life had not been very supportive during her childhood years. She had spent most of her leisure time in the house while her divorced mother worked. She was anxious to leave as soon as she graduated from special classes in high school. She saw marriage as the only way out and pursued that option. Following Carl's death she recognized her need to have fun and that she could not meet her children's needs at the same time. She therefore placed them in foster care. Betty's situation leads to the question of how permission to see other options and limited information and suggestions to her mother regarding her need for adolescent self-expression might have prevented her early marriage and childbearing.

In two of the couples who married early, a history of severe family problems including divorce and child and/or sexual abuse co-existed with learning problems. It therefore seems likely that all of the above might not have worked without intensive therapy.

Despite intensive therapy for both herself and her family during her teenage years, Rachel chose marriage as the way out of a difficult family situation.

Rachel and Charles were the first couple I treated in premarital counselling. The importance of involving family and dealing with the issue of family relations was poignantly learned through this case. Rachel, anxious to please, agreed to move to Phoenix along with her mother-in-law, who had indicated in my one contact with her that she had no intention of asking "the children" to make the move. The isolation from friends and family was a major source of the depression and frustration that led Rachel to divorce.

These situations lead us to ask ourselves what happens if the marriage fails? Here again the clinician can call upon the permission-giving and limited information approaches in working with clients and families. Permission to fail and to experience the dignity of risk (Perske 1972) is important. Families often ask the clinician to guarantee that their child will succeed in independent living or marriage. Since such guarantees are impossible for those *without* learning problems, it appears even more remote for developmentally disabled couples.

Our role then must be to provide permission to families to see their anxieties as normal, but to give information about the need for risk-taking to promote growth. To the couple themselves, the clinician will hopefully be able to provide permission to exercise the right to risk-taking, and at the same time, information about the particular risks which may jeopardize marital functioning. This is especially difficult while preventing our biases from surfacing. Based upon the experience of the couples in my group, I have learned to counsel couples coming for premarital therapy about the problems which may arise over the question of family visits. This has been important in counselling June and Donald.

June and Donald have known each other for a little over a year. Both are participating in an independent living project and plan to marry as soon as they can save enough money for the deposit on an apartment. Neither of their parents approve of the marriage. Donald's father rarely sees him anymore. June's parents spend time with her and have her home for weekends, but refuse to have Donald along. Donald feels badly about this. June feels badly about leaving him, but wants to see her family. In this case, I have attempted to give both of them permission to see their feelings as normal. I have provided them with information about the kind of problems this kind of situation has caused other couples after marriage. Specific suggestions have focused on ways to help Donald express his feelings about this and help June talk to her parents about her wish to have Donald included in her visits.

What if things do not work out and there are disagreements? I have found myself doing much pre- and post-marital counselling around the normalcy and even desirability of disagreements in a relationship, taking into account the risks of allowing these to escalate into violence. The right to a less-than-perfect relationship has been an important area for permission-giving. Information about the existence of disagreement in most relationships has been necessary to combat fantasties of marriage without conflict and fears about disaster if disagreements occur. This has been most relevant for June and Donald. Both believed that marriage should be totally without strife and point to histories of strife in their own families and of experiencing abuse at the hands of their parents.

After an argument, they were both devastated and several times Donald got up on the roof of the apartment and threatened to jump. When frustrated with problems of communication, both have resorted to physical violence. In pre-marital counselling, we are engaged in all four levels of approach: permission to have disagreements and see them as a normal part of the relationship, information about the risks of using physical aggression or threats to solve them, and specific suggestions around better ways to problem solve disagreements as well as intensive therapy focusing on individual and conjoint issues.

In counselling families, I often hear of their concerns that the couple will be unable to keep an apartment up to standard. When I describe students who rent small apartments and their often deplorable standard of housekeeping, the usual response is that they are busy studying. Again and again I am confronted with the phenomenon of higher expectation for disabled people. Somehow, college students' sloppiness is blamed on their studying, while for the developmentally disabled couple it is blamed on their learning problems and intellectual limitations.

Must a relationship be perfect to be attempted? Must a person be able to function independently, meeting "middle class" standards for housekeeping and appearance? Clinicians and families alike must ask themselves whether they can accept less than perfect functioning and give themselves and clients and their families permission to accept this as well.

Often the clinician will find a relationship so imperfect that he or she will question why the couple wants to stay together. For several of the couples I have assisted, the answer has to do with what they see as a lack of alternatives. Marriage has afforded them independence, and for most, believing that they could not make it on their own, they feel that divorce would mean a return home. In marriage, in spite of all the difficulties, they have found companionship. Companionship is almost uniformlly given as the most important reason for marrying among couples interviewed by myself, Janet Mattinson (1975), and the Crafts (1979).

Bill epitomizes this feeling:

> I find we have companionship. We do things of interest together. I mean and, un, I'm not lonely anymore. I mean, I have a good job and my job works out much better nowadays, since I've been married. I mean I can go to work and I feel good and all that and I have someone to come home to and I feel I have a much better life now.[3]

I have been impressed with the longevity of the marriages I have seen, in spite of great interpersonal and external stresses. It has been interesting to watch the demise of several very recent marriages of four years or less duration. The ever increasing divorce rate and its acceptance as normal may have an impact on couples with developmental disabilities, but we can only speculate on this.

Counselling couples experiencing severe stress employs all levels of approach; some times it centres around permission to express unhappiness, but still remain married; sometimes information regarding options is given when the going gets particularly rough (board-and-care, sharing an apartment); also, divorce may be considered and specific suggestions and intensive therapy to improve the relationship may be provided.

Group Counselling

Much of the postmarital counselling has been done in the group setting. A discussion of the methods used would take up an entire chapter in itself. The group modality cannot be recommended too highly. It provides the dimensions of peer support and feedback. As others have noted, those with handicaps may be the best help to others who share their problems (Craft and Craft 1979). Often, I have found members able to accept the negative feedback from their peers which they would have rejected from others. I believe that educational and vocational advances made by many members would not have occurred without the support of their peers. There is also the therapeutic effect of relating an experience or feeling and knowing the listener has been there too.

Our therapeutic tools have centred around a series of mainly behavioural and experiential techniques. We have employed assertion training and behavioural marital therapy techniques. We also have made extensive use of role play methods with video feedback whenever possible (Liberman *et al* 1975 and 1980).

Our group sessions have tended to move rather freely through all levels of the PLISSIT model. At times we will be giving one couple or partner permission to feel good or bad about something that has already happened, or permission to express feelings previously held within. Often this will take the form of one partner receiving the group's support for his or her expression of needs to the other.

Often a session will be spent providing information, usually from member to member rather than from the therapists. This will often centre around questions of employment, family relations, or dealings with various government agencies. Occasionally we will invite a speaker on a relevant topic.

Sometimes the information given is in the form of feedback, about how they appear to others or what effect their behaviour may be having. This usually escalates to the point of intensive therapy, and issues of group process come to the fore. Because of the long-term nature and support function of the group as well as the outside friendships which have developed, the general therapeutic process is less intense than that characteristic of shorter term groups.

Counselling Concerns

Procreation: Counselling concerning procreation has been my most challenging and difficult experience. The dignity of risk and the right to attempt things though they may turn out imperfect becomes problematic when they involve the life of a child. The clinician has very limited information at his disposal regarding the ability or lack of it of developmentally disabled couples to parent.

Where the specific question asked is whether there is a chance of hereditary retardation, genetic counselling is available. The state of the art is such, however, that there are definite answers in only a few cases. For most, as in Rachel's case, there is a guess, a supposition. For others, the answer is even less clear.

On the issue of child-bearing, we must ask whether anyone in society has the right to grant or revoke permission for another person to procreate. We cannot force abortion upon those known to be carrying deformed fetuses. For that matter, we do not terminate the right to procreate of those who have abused or even murdered their children. In the practice of pre- and post-marital counselling with this population the clinician is often asked to be party to denying the right to procreate, usually by being involved in decisions regarding sterilization. When counselling couples and their families, it is important that the clinician provides information about the difference between deciding against sterilization and deciding to have children. A decision not to bear children can be a time limited one with the possibility of change if life circumstances change. A decision to be sterilized has life-long implications. Giving couples correct information about sterilization and the risks of having handicapped children is not concomitant with suggesting they have children. Information and specific suggestions about birth control methods can be provided. The clinician must provide information about the costs and responsibilities of parenthood and the potential problems. This two-sided counselling situation is well illustrated by Kay and Jeremy.

When Kay and Jeremy had been married less than a year, she found herself pregnant. Her family and his father were alarmed and counselled strongly against having the child. The professionals working with them attempted to be objective. In the realm of permission giving, they counselled Kay as to her rights to make the final decision and, also, provided information both about abortions and the realities of parenting at this stage in their marriage. They brought their dilemma to a couples' group meeting as well. Their peers provided much information about their own child-bearing and raising experiences. Those who were childless counselled against Kay allowing herself to have the sterilization her mother was suggesting should happen at the time of the abortion. They also spoke of her rights to make her own decision. Ultimately, Kay and Jeremy were able to use all this input to decide not to have a child at this time but not to permanently terminate their ability to procreate.

In the same way, the clinician working with couples and families in the pre-marital stage must help them to see that issues of marriage and parenthood are also separate. Many couples who accept their own inability to raise children are enjoying being married. Several families I have seen opposed marriage on the grounds that they did not want to take care of the potential grandchildren. If the couple has decided not to have children, helping the family see the separation between marriage and parenthood may help them resolve their oppositional feelings. Where the couple insists upon having children, the situation becomes more complicated. The clinician is then called upon to provide information about the separateness of the two decisions and suggest that perhaps they deal with the issue of marriage and postpone the decision to have children through the use of birth control. This question arose with June and Donald.

> Both June and Donald want to have children and see sexual relations as clearly to accomplish this end. However, in order to obtain his father's support for his move to an independent living project, Donald agreed to a vasectomy. Early in pre-marital counselling they asked for information about reversal operations and adoption. They were aware that they did not want to have children right away but saw this as the expression of marriage, and therefore the most vital to discuss. With permission to hold this hope for the future, but with information about the need to get genetic counselling due to June's seizure disorder, they have been able to focus on the more immediate financial, communication, and familial issues confronting them.

The clinician working with younger children and their families can play an important role as well. Early messages saying that child-rearing is not the only method of self-fulfillment, especially for women, are urgently needed. We must remember to alert parents that this will be a most difficult message to convey because only a very small portion of the population does *not* see child-bearing as normative, and the cultural pressure on people to procreate is enormous.

Sexual Pleasure: If sexuality is not just for making babies, then what *is* it for? Herein lies the challenge to professionals involved in education and counselling settings, with young children and their families, as well as with adults. The roots of prevention of sexual dysfunction also lie in the provision of early messages. What messages are usually given to developmentally disabled individuals at the outset about such things as touch, pleasure, positive body image, existence as a sexual being? What message is conveyed to the teenager dressed in outdated and over-sized clothes about his sexuality? How often is the retarded child rewarded for his cute and affectionate behaviour towards others, and the same retarded teenager over-sheltered for fear of exploitation due to over-friendliness?

Clinicians involved with young children and their families are obliged to provide them with information about the long-term effects of their early messages. For sexuality to become a source of pleasure, a form of communication, an expression of relationship, we must give positive messages from the earliest opportunity. We must give families specific suggestions about how they can help their child learn to value and care for their own bodies. We must provide them with correct information about such things as masturbation, correcting old myths, so that they can teach this to their own children. We must give them specific suggestions on how to respond to such things as finding their child masturbating.

Thus, we may avoid the sexual fears expressed by several of our couples, centring round negative responses to masturbation and nakedness as children. These have found expression in adulthood in the inability to be naked together, or to touch themselves in any way in the presence of the partner.

Sex Education: It is in the provision of sex education and the development of curricula that most clinicians and educators can make an impact on the sexual functioning of future marriages within this population.

Most of the sexuality education these couples received in the past centred around the issues of prevention of pregnancy and birth control. Sexuality has been presented as intercourse within the context of a unit on human reproduction. For those fearful of pregnancy or veneral disease, this has led to phobic responses regarding sexual contact. On a more general level, it has supported scripted messages regarding sexuality as equal to intercourse which is then equal to procreation and to responses such as Caroline's: "Sexual intercourse is a necessary evil if you want to have children." And Robin's, "My husband says why bother to have sex if you aren't going to try to get pregnant?" For those already determined to have a child, pictures of pretty babies coupled with talk of intercourse have only reinforced their desire.

I would propose an alternate model of sex education which would focus on a broader range of methods to derive pleasure from sensuality and sexuality. For instance, can we teach about the sensuality of hand, foot, face, and full body caress? Can we stress that not everyone has intercourse every time there is sex play?

Crucial information to be provided includes such things as: what is a female orgasm; the differing rates of the sexual response cycle in men and women, the fact that lubrication is only the beginning of the woman's sexual response cycle and does not mean the vagina is ready for penetration (this seems to account for much of the pain women describe); that all men experience transient erectile failures, that it is normal for the man to be unable to regain an erection for a period of time after ejaculating (refractory periods); about the importance of the clitoris in triggering female orgasm; that in the case of sexual relations speed is not necessarily desirable; the necessity to seek help if they find themselves unable to ejaculate; and about such things as the necessary stimulation required for orgasm and the need for thrusting.

Specific suggestions will usually fall within the purview of the counsellor rather than the educator. However, assignments such as looking at one's body and identifying things that one likes and does not like about it could be integrated into sex education programmes as well as counselling. A valuable impact can also be made through the teaching of communication skills. Role playing can be valuable in teaching a person to ask for and turn down or postpone sexual advances made by a partner. A hand massage exercise can be used to teach ways of communicating positive messages.

Those involved in counselling couples both before and after marriage can have a significant effect on sexual functioning and possibly help prevent the development of dysfunctions requiring intensive therapy. Much important work can be done on the levels of permission, limited information and specific suggestions. All the couples I have seen required permission to see the sexual aspects of the relationship as potential sources of pleasure, and to accept self-pleasuring and nudity as normal.

Perhaps the most important area of permission-giving has been in feeling that the problems they experience are not so different from the so-called normal population. Several of the couples I have treated have been pleased to know that other sex therapy patients, some with professional backgrounds, do not always know where the clitoris is or that women do not ejaculate on orgasm. All this is education in its widest sense.

Much of the same information provided in sexuality education needs to be repeated in counselling. Couples can also benefit from a series of specific suggestions. I have found instructions in Sensate Focus to be most helpful. The reader is directed to a series of films on this and other techniques available from RDCOA.[4] A major area in which we can provide specific suggestions is communication. Counsellors can model and have couples practice ways both to initiate and accept or reject their partners' sexual advances. Specific suggestions about more effective methods of stimulation or ways to integrate the use of various birth control methods into the course of love-making are often necessary.

Approach to Sexual Problems: Assessing the couples' specific problems can pose quite a challenge. Here again, I have found the use of slides and other visual aids helpful. Viewing a slide of a man masturbating in the "average" way allowed Jeremy to explain that during his years in boarding school, he had learned to masturbate by rubbing himself against the rug while fully clothed. This explained why he did not understand instructions regarding the use of a stop-start technique for premature ejaculation predicated upon manual stimulation. In Donald's case, complaints of pain upon intercourse were unclear. Showing slides of circumcised and uncircumcised penises allowed him to illustrate a problem he was having with the foreskin, and suggestions were made about the necessary hygiene to solve the difficulty.

Perhaps the most important thing in counselling is to follow the adage NEVER ASSUME ANYTHING. I am constantly reminded by my work with these couples that they use words which do not always convey what they mean and often do not reveal the whole scope of a problem at once. Careful assessment is vital.

Another cautionary note from my experience is that suggestions such as exaggerating a body part that you do not like for purposes of desensitization (sticking out your stomach, etc.) is regarded as a putdown, whereas average couples often find it helpful. Also any materials which depict handicapped people (such as the film "Touching") have been seen as a statement suggesting that I felt they were cripples. By the same token, satirical films, such as *Quickie,* have been accepted as the gospel. Richard said, "That

283

must be the way it should be, or you wouldn't show it to us and also it's the way it has to be because we have to finish before George and Laurie [the couple that shares their apartment in a board and care home] walk in."

Need for Intensive Therapy: Many couples will require intensive sexual dysfunction therapy in spite of all the efforts of the counsellor. For the provision of such therapy, intensive training is required. Readers are advised to contact human sexuality programmes in large universities regarding training and resources.

Conclusion

The work I have done with these couples has left an indelible impression. The hours spent with them has been time well used in terms of personal-professional satisfaction and growth. I hope others will develop an interest in service to this group and will find my experience instructive and that those already involved will have gained something as well.

NOTES

(1) Sec. 102: A developmental disability is a severe, chronic disability attributed to a mental and/or physical impairment, manifested before the person reaches age 22, which is likely to continue indefinitely, and which:
  (a) Results in substantial functional limitation in *three or more* of the following areas of major life activity:
      self care   receptive and expressive language
      learning
      mobility   capacity for independent living
      self-direction
      economic sufficiency
  (b) Reflects the person's need for a combination of individually planned and coordinated care, treatment or other services which are of extended duration.
(2) In *Handicapped Married Couples,* Ann and Michael Craft describe a population composed of persons whose IQs are below 70 and therefore labelled mentally handicapped and a group with higher IQs labelled personality disordered.
(3) *With This Ring I Thee Wed,* Videotape, produced by UCLA, Mental Retardation Child Psychiatry Program, 760 Westwood Plaza, Los Angeles, California 90024.
(4) Current regulations for the use of federal funds in sterilization—Department of Health and Human Services, U.S. Government.
(5) EDCOA Production, Inc., 310 Cedar Lane, Teaneck, New Jersey 07666.

REFERENCES

Regarding marriage, parenthood and birth control among developmentally disabled couples

Andron, L. and Sturm, M.L. (1973). Is "I do" in the Repertoire of the Retarded? *Ment.Retardaton 11,* 31–4.

Craft, A. and Craft, M. (1979). *Handicapped Married Couples.* London and Boston: Routledge and Kegan Paul.

Craft, M. and Craft, A. (1978). *Sex and the Mentally Handicapped.* London and Boston: Routledge and Kegan Paul.

Mattinson, J. (1975). *Marriage and Mental Handicap.* London: Institute of Marital Studies, The Tavistock Institute of Human Relations. Second edition.

Perske, R. (1972). The Dignity of Risk and the Mentally Retarded. *Ment.Retardation 10,* 1, 25–7.

Sabagh, C. and Edgerton, R.B. (1962). Sterilized Mental Defectives look at Eugenic Sterilization. *Eugenics Quarterly 9,* 4, 213–22.

References regarding sexual dysfunction and therapy

Annon, J.S. (1974). *The Behavioral Treatment of Sexual Problems,* Vol. I *Brief Therapy.* Honolulu: Enabling Systems.

Barbach, L.G. (1976). *For Yourself: The fulfillment of female sexuality.* New York: Anchor Press/Doubleday.

Frank, E., Anderson, C. and Rubinstein, D. (1978). Frequency of sexual dysfunction in "normal" couples. *New England Journal of Medicine 299,* 111.

Gagon, J. (1977). *Human Sexualities.* Glenview, Ill.: Scott, Foresman.

Heinman, J., LoPiccolo, L. and LoPiccolo, J. (1976). *Becoming Orgasmic: A sexual growth program for women.* New Jersey: Prentice-Hall.

Hite, S. (1976). *The Hite report.* New York: Dell.

Hunt, J. (1974). *Sexual behavior in the 1970's.* New York: Dell.

Kaplan, H.S. (1974). *The New Sex Therapy: Active treatment of sexual dysfunctions.* New York: Quadrangle/The New York Times Book Co.

Kolodny, C., Masters, W.H. and Johnson, V.E. (1979). *Textbook of Sexual Medicine.* Boston: Little Brown and Co.

Lobitz, W.C. and LoPiccolo, J. (1972). New methods in the behavioral treatment of sexual dysfunction. *Journal of Behavior Therapy and Experimental Psychiatry, 3,* 265–71.

LoPiccolo, J. (1978). Direct treatment of sexual dysfunction. In: LoPiccolo, J. and LoPiccolo, L. (eds.) *Handbook of Sex Therapy.* New York: Plenum Press.

Masters, W.H. and Johnson, V.E. (1966). *Human Sexual Response.* Boston: Little, Brown and Co.

Masters, W.H. and Johnson, V.E. (1970). *Human Sexual Inadequacy.* Boston: Little, Brown and Co.

Masters, W.H. and Johnson, V.E. (1979). Homosexuality in Perspective. Boston: Little, Brown and Co.

Price, S., Golden, J.S., Golden, M., Price, T., Heinrich, A.G. and Munford, P. (1978). Training family planning personnel in sex counseling and sex education. *Public Health Reports 93,* 328–34.

Task Force on Concerns of Physically Disabled Women (1978). *Toward Intimacy.* New York: Human Sciences Press. (Reproductive Health Services, 1507 21st Street, Suite 100, Sacramento Ca. 95814.)

Ziegler, F.J. (1970). Vasectomy and Adverse Psychological Reactions. *Annals of Internal Medicine, 73,* 853.

285

References regarding technique

Brown, J. (1979). *Back to the Beanstalk*. La Jolla: Psychology and Consulting Associates Press.

Jacobson, N. and Margolin, G. (1979). *Marital Therapy: Strategies based on social and behavior exchange principles*. New York: Bruner/Mazel.

Liberman, R., Wheeler, E.. de Visser, L., Kuehnel, J. and Knelvel, T. (1980). *Handbook of Marital Therapy: A Positive Approach to Helping Troubled Relationships*. New York: Plenum Press.

Liberman, R., King, L., De Risi, W.J. and McCann, M.J. (1975). *Personal Effectiveness: Guiding People to Assert Themselves and Improve their Social Skills*. Champaign: Research Press.

Simon, S.B., Howe, L.W. and Kirschenbaum H. (1972). *Values Clarification: A Handbook of Practical Strategies*. New York: Hart Publishing.

CHAPTER 13

An International Perspective

Victoria Shennan

No appraisal of international practice in the education of mentally handicapped people can be attempted without using the Declaration of Rights of the Retarded, adopted in 1971 by the General Assembly of the United Nations as a yardstick. Nor can it be forgotten that the first statement of that Declaration is that mentally retarded people have the same basic rights of other citizens of the same country and same age. (United Nations 1971).

It follows that no evaluation of practices anywhere in the world can be made without relevance to the provision of such education for all citizens, and the understanding that these provisions will be made on the basis of local needs, within local resources and in line with historical, cultural and social factors prevalent in those countries.

However excellent programmes may prove in their country of origin it is unlikely that they will transfer outside it with total success. All the more reason, then, to examine the *principles* which dictate our own practices, to compare them with experience elsewhere and to be ready to change and modify ideas in line with changing conditions.

The Declaration concludes with what is perhaps the most important part of these rights, 'the right to respect', and therefore of their recognition as members of the human family, wherever they may live. The acceptance of mentally handicapped people as neighbours entitled to live alongside others and to share equally the amenities of community life depends to a very great extent on the way mentally handicapped people have previously been regarded by that society; the factors which are affecting a change of attitude; and the speed of that change.

Nowhere is this seen more clearly than in changing attitudes to sexuality, marriage, family life and family breakdown, and the speed of these changes sometimes invokes a rapid reaction against previous values, or an increased determination to withstand pressures to change.

287

In the United Kingdom, the past thirty years have seen a revolution in public attitudes to sexuality. A whole area of human personality, hitherto almost totally beset by taboos and secrecy, emerged suddenly into the fields of public view, public discussion and overt display.

That so much attention is still focussed on sexuality in its more erotic manifestations may be an indicator of a continued uncertainty of the place of sexual relationships within society as a whole. The debates upon the relative roles of the sexes, contraception, abortion, exploitation of women as sex objects, the equal sharing of the parent role by husband and wife, all point to a period of constant change and appraisal which is unlikely to be quickly resolved.

The dramatic change from hidden sexual activity to a totally open attitude has left many people completely confused. Intellectually, they accept as rational the view that sexuality is a facet of the whole human personality which should be able to be considered as objectively and rationally as the rest of life. Emotionally, they are assailed by completely different reactions, and these powerfully affect their attitudes to the sexual life of others, particularly the handicapped.

Some mentally handicapped adults, both men and women, appear to have an instinctive feeling that the sexual area of their lives is an area of privacy. One sees this also in children approaching puberty who are required to listen to sexual education from adults. Sometimes parents are rebuffed when they wish to open such a discussion, especially if there has been no ease of communication earlier. Professionals involved with mentally handicapped people may meet with a similar withdrawl of attention if they initiate discussion. This urge to privacy in sexual relations may stem from primitive practical experience that the human couple are at their most vulnerable during the act of intercourse. If this had not been generally carried out in security, free from the danger of attack or other violence, the human race could not have long survived. Whatever the explanation, the instinctive desire for privacy in the whole area of sexuality needs to be understood and respected when programmes are being designed for mentally handicapped people, no less than others.

The new freedom of expression sometimes has the effect of an over-reaction by some non-mentally handicapped adults. It can be seen in the desire by some creative people to test the limits of public acceptance of personal attitudes in literature, films and television for example. In its turn, such personal displays may produce an equally violent reaction from those who tenaciously hold different views. What may be overlooked is that demands for special rights for *any* group of people, by alienating public opinion, may in fact have the result of depriving that group of facilities and services available to all, because undue attention has been drawn to the differences of the group, rather than on the common human needs shared by everyone.

In any country, public opinions and attitudes at local and national level precede statutory regulations, and form the base for legislation or provisions which will be acceptable to the society involved. In addition, increased speed of communication world-wide influences reactions to change within one country by awareness of the results of change elsewhere.

All programmes of integration from the family into community life require the active participation of the parents of mentally handicapped children and adolescents if they are to succeed.

For all parents, the time of preparation of children to leave the family is a period of anxiety and stress; both child and parent are re-evaluating their roles and view the future in the world outside with anticipation and fear. The doubts and uncertainties of young adults may result in aggressive behaviour towards parental restrictions hitherto accepted. If these are openly expressed some resolution is possible but, when a communication difficulty exists, particularly if there is a problem of inadequate vocabulary to express the emotions experienced, the period of preparing to leave home can be traumatic for both parent and child, and may only be resolved when the new situation has also emerged from the unstable phase into a more settled condition.

The process of adapting to change may be short or long, depending upon past experience and the personality of the individual. It cannot be hurried. The trial of a new home situation for mentally handicapped people will need time and patience and the willingness to examine the reasons for difficulty and the courage to commence afresh after a failure.

The teaching must commence with the early understanding of social behaviour in general, of respect for the opinions of others and their desire to live happily in society by acceptance of social customs which may not always be those the individual would choose for

289

himself. Such teaching is an essential part of the education of mentally handicapped children and needs to be introduced at the earliest moment.

Because of his limited mental capacity, the child will not be able to select from the patterns of behaviour around him and to understand the risks of deviant patterns. His comprehension of cause and effect will be limited to actual experience and so new situations will find him unprepared. He cannot easily transfer learning from one situation to another and by predicting the consequences evaluate the risks.

If a good family life, the sharing of the joys and sorrows with a small group of like-minded people, is a desirable end, it is best prepared for by that way of life by example. People who have been denied this experience because of years spent in institutions from childhood have an enormous task to learn new attitudes appropriate to life in the community. In simple skills of housekeeping, shopping, using public services and of social contacts, particularly those relating to sexuality, they have no pattern to follow and so need patient support as they learn to live with friends in the small group home. Opportunities to observe how harmonious relationships are created by compromise are learnt early in family life and absorbed unconsciously into a pattern, which may later be rejected, but which nevertheless conditions future attitudes.

Staff faced with preparing patients to leave hospitals for community life may be faced with teaching adults with no experience whatever of family life, as ignorant of the roles of parents, the extended family and of friends and neighbours as if they had dropped from another planet.

Years of ignorance cannot be quickly made up, but now that the problem is recognised, original and innovative methods of teaching are increasingly being used.

The current BBC Television series of *Let's Go* has selected several areas of family living—entertaining friends, decorating a room to personal taste, choosing suitable clothing—and presents them at a pace which enables the practical points made to be fully understood, whilst ensuring that social attitudes are equally well observed. Such preparation is a necessary pre-requisite to the introduction of more specific instruction for family and sexual life.

EUROPE

Education

The right of mentally handicapped people to share fully in community life means that preparation for such a life style must include education in sexual behaviour, marriage and parenthood and the need for, and means of, controlled family planning. Preparation for family life is an integral part of education and sex education, a part of the whole of life. It follows that, just as the ordinary subjects of literacy and numeracy may need special programmes of study and will certainly need more prolonged and repetitive work, so the same degree of patience and an individual approach will be needed, if mentally handicapped young adults are to leave educational courses properly prepared.

United Kingdom

In the United Kingdom, funds for education are provided by the state and administered by the Local Education Authority. The curriculum is not centrally laid down, but is usually dictated by the demands of the examining boards who will be responsible for the examinations taken by pupils as they leave the school system. It follows, therefore, that education for sexual life and preparation for family life in the community will vary from school to school and from area to area. Local education committees will interpret the responsibility for teaching within all their schools with strong local bias. This will reflect the local attitudes, which vary a great deal according to geographic, social and economic factors.

Mentally handicapped young adults may remain within the school system until the age of nineteen years, and may have some link with the further and adult education provisions later, through attendance at an Adult Training Centre.

Many Adult Training Centres have been greatly concerned with the need to give some basic education in sexual matters to the young people who attend their centres (Lowes 1977; Cumbria Social Services Dept., undated). Crisis situations develop during the working day which require immediate action upon the part of the staff.

However, when the young adult is over 18 years of age, the parent is no longer the natural guardian. In the absence of a formal legal

291

ruling to the contrary, the mentally handicapped young adult is responsible for his own actions. Staff and instructors at ATC's are therefore not acting in *loco parentis* for adults over this age, but find themselves in the invidious situation of being responsible to their employing authority for the welfare of their trainees, and challenged by the parents of those who are still living at home if they undertake tasks which the parents see as beyond their duty.

Many authorities have had excellent co-operation with parents and with the staff of hostels and hospitals which are the residence of their trainees, and undoubtedly this is to the benefit of all.

Sweden

Sweden has long been in the forefront of projects of education and preparation for adult life for the mentally handicapped.

The Swedish Institute produces fact sheets on the trends within the country and the February 1980 edition makes a significant statement on the concept of handicap. The approach 'shifts the handicap from the individuals to their environment' and places a responsibility on the public to make amenities accessible. Though the statement relates to physical handicap, the philosophy is clear— normalisation means giving access to all aspects of life to all citizens. It is this attitude which has enabled Karl Grunewald to develop his work on liberating mentally handicapped people from the closed, institutionalised environment into the open community, with full participation in family life. (Grunewald 1979; Grunewald and Linner 1979.)

There are no longer formal obstacles to marriage by mentally handicapped people, only the one which applies to other citizens, that they must fully comprehend the contract to which they subscribe. In past years up to 1940, Sweden had a compulsory sterilisation law designed to restrict the conception of children by mentally handicapped people.

Karl Grunewald regards as an essential prerequisite to efficient mothering, the experience of satisfying emotional contacts with her own mother in childhood, a conclusion now generally accepted for all. He recommends a firm network of support for a mentally handicapped mother to ensure a good pattern for the child, and above all, that adequate sexual advice and counselling should commence in the early teens, and that mentally handicapped young women should participate in the programmes of training for motherhood provided for other young women in the community.

Though mentally handicapped people are less likely to be parents than others in the same age group, the contacts with other young women will enable the mentally handicapped girl to understand attitudes and to be aware of current trends.

He states that in Sweden the experience has been fewer births to mentally handicapped women in the past decade than ever before and attributes this to the programmes of education, and advice on contraception.

Netherlands

In Holland stress is laid upon the fact that the education of mentally handicapped children is part of a whole philosophy of special education, which embraces all handicapped children. The aim is to prepare pupils as far as possible to lead their own lives in society and not to depend on others. Programmes are based upon the individual capabilities of each child, but there is a clear statement that children who will always be dependent upon others—the profoundly handicapped—are dependent upon nursing. The profoundly handicapped are prepared through the school age years for sheltered workshop employment and receive support and guidance from the instructional staff.

The multi-disciplinary teams who have supported the child at school, teachers, psychologists, doctors and social workers, will continue to be a resource when the adolescent leaves school. Many pupils return to their old school for advice and help with problems which arise, even many years after leaving school.

The whole curriculum is centrally controlled and there is an agency entitled 'Specialised Work with Young People and Adults' (GJVW) which provides courses designed to bridge the various leisure and social agencies existing and to co-ordinate their efforts.

The National Federation of Social Services for the Mentally Handicapped administers a compulsory in-service advanced training programme for social workers who are employed by the social work services. Centrally agreed policy is therefore practically implemented.

Government funded Day Centres and Sheltered Workshops have

a long experience and excellent reputation and voluntary organisations receive government subsidy for approved projects.

Belgium

Belgium has special institutes for handicapped children and adults and the programmes are individually designed according to the needs and abilities of those concerned, and state education is provided for mentally handicapped people up to secondary level.

Attitudes to sexual education follow the liberal European pattern: as in Holland, education for sexual life is seen as part of a whole, and segregation of the sexes in residential situations is not practised.

NORTH AMERICA

In the United States until recently, public education has been the responsibility of each state government. Each State has a department of special education. Recently the federal government has increased its role in education, particularly in the field of equal opportunity and has initiated the Office of Special Education and Rehabilitation Services in the Washington Department of Education. The Office has a specific duty for both mentally and physically handicapped students. Since 1976 the Education for All Handicapped Children Act has required states receiving Federal Aid to provide specially designed programmes for handicapped pupils. These programmes include vocational training, counselling and physical therapy to enable them to obtain employment. Such programmes, administered by the Office of Special Education and Rehabilitation Services, will vary from state to state.

In general, the facilities available to other young adults, including preparation for marrying and parenthood which are normally given at 13-14 years, are available to mentally handicapped young people with the additional provision, already established, of programmes designed for individual needs. It is possible that the approach to such teaching is more direct and objective than in the United Kingdom, and reflects the particular qualities and attitudes of the American nation as a whole.

The National Society for Mentally Handicapped Children and Adults has used some American-made film programmes on sexual education for mentally handicapped young adults for some time to stimulate discussion. These films have aroused great interest when they are shown and reveal clearly the difference in approach by one particular American teacher from those in more general use in the United Kingdom.

There are a number of voluntary organisations throughout the United States providing education and services for mentally handicapped people, some of these include group counselling, health and hygiene, social and personal relationships, instruction within their post school assessment and training projects. Some of these provide group homes and training for mentally handicapped young adults to live in them.

CANADA

In Canada, education is the responsibilty of individual provincial governments and the programmes provided in each will be different. There is no centrally agreed curriculum on sexual education in the schools and in Quebec province, for example, there is a special education service of the Ministry of Education which advises on all aspects of curriculum content.

For non-communicating mentally handicapped people a system, Blissymbolics was perfected in Toronto and a programme of sex education, using the Bliss symbols, has been designed by Frederick Lapham (1980). It attempts to describe intercourse and possible reproduction in the simplest possible terms and is another example of the wide range of programmes currently exploring this field.

AUSTRALIA

In Australia the settlers came from a wide variety of countries, and early attempts to follow the British systems of state education linked to the established church were soon challenged. A dual system emerged, with a Denominational Board administering educational funds for those schools offering Church of England religious instruction, and a national board which administered the funds for schools for all, regardless of denomination. It is possible that the widespread provision of educational facilities by voluntary bodies is a result of this situation, an inevitable consequence of the acceptance of varied needs, and of geographic features which make the local provisions imperative.

Many provisions for education for mentally handicapped children are substantially supported by voluntary effort. Teachers may be provided by government, but premises and equipment may be totally funded by local groups. This situation makes participation by parents much more acceptable, and preparation for family life more likely.

Sexual attitudes, however, will materially affect the content of this teaching. As recently as January 6th 1981, the Australian Express reported that the Concerned Parents' Association in Melbourne—an association not concerned with the mentally handicapped—has raised a large sum of money and acquired 500 members to campaign against uninhibited sex education in schools in Victoria. Such attitudes cannot be ignored. Provisions for mentally handicapped citizens cannot be regarded in isolation. In Queensland more conservative attitudes are seen in other situations. The January 1981 edition of *Penthouse* was banned in Brisbane and the magazine will not in future be allowed into the state. Voluntary schools for mentally handicapped young people with government teachers have additional problems in the north of the state where many pupils come from rural communities and from wide social and ethnic backgrounds. The few Aboriginal children we saw attending a school in Cairns, Queensland would return to their tribal situations where the sexual attitudes would be dictated by the vanishing remnants of centuries old practices.

This Centre had a major transport problem. Widely scattered as the rural community is, a good part of each day is spent in the bus which brings them to the Centre. At least by spending the weekends in their own community the children were maintaining a link with the family life there. The importance of a harmonious relationship with parents and an agreement on the content of all educational programmes was well understood, and parent participation in the centres was close.

DEVELOPING COUNTRIES

Mental handicap is prevalent throughout the world and is a reminder that all men are brothers. Dr B. W. Richards, lately consultant psychiatrist at St Lawrence's Hospital, Caterham has spent a lifetime studying genetic factors in mental handicap, in particular Down's anomaly, and has a collection of slide photographs of people suffering from this condition from all ethnic groups, eskimo, indian, african, south american and caucasian.

The term, 'Third world countries', is in itself divisive. There is only one world, which we all share, and if we value intelligence and the mastery of advanced technologies above other human values we are in danger of losing the balance provided by the essential qualities of compassion and humanity which distinguish mankind.

We have an enormous fund of knowledge, as a result of scientific advances, but we still lack the wisdom needed to make the best use of it. The pattern of life in the industrialised countries is all too often considered as a desirable state for all countries, our missionary activities have left the field of religion and entered those of science and in particular, of medicine, sometimes with disastrous results.

We need to remember that we suffer today in the United Kingdom from an inheritance of past wrong thinking, our huge mental handicap hospitals are but one example, and that we have perhaps as much to learn from the developing countries of the world as they from us. We need the reminder that communication involves listening as well as talking and the International League Congress in Nairobi in 1982 has declared as its first objective 'Reaching out *from* developing countries to other nations'.

In 1972, Dr Lambo, Assistant Director General of the World Health Organization, speaking at a Conference mounted by the Royal Society of Health described a training programme for people who were mentally disabled, centred upon rural villages in remote districts south of the Sahara. He was asked whether his practices, designed for such conditions, would be workable in industrial areas. His reply was 'We know that our *methods* may not be appropriate and may become obsolete, but we are trying to discover which conditions benefit these people, and to derive a *philosophy* which will translate to other environments and help them there'.

Such a philosophy may well have universal application; we must not forget to observe carefully how problems such as those presented by the philosophy of normalisation and of fulfilment of sexuality are translated into practice in other countries, and not be so concerned with exporting our ideas that we fail to import those which may be of great value as we define our own objectives.

REFERENCES

Cumbria Social Services Dept. (undated). *Health and Sex Education Programme.* Mill Lane Adult Training Centre.

Grunewald, K. (1979). Sex Liberation and Parenthood for the Mentally Retarded in Sweden. Paper published by Socialstyrelsen, the National Board of Health and Welfare, 106 30 Stockholm, Sweden, July 1979.

Grunewald, K. and Linner, B. (1979). Mentally Retarded: Sexuality and Normaliation. *Current Sweden* No 237, Dec. 1979.

Lambo, T.A. (1972). Health and Social Services for the Mentally Handicapped. Address given at the Royal Society of Health Conference, Isle of Man, 6th September, 1972.

Lapham, F.G. (1980). *Life Begins.* Toronto: Blissymbolics Communication Institute.

Lowes, L. (1977). *Sex and Social Training.* London: NSMHC.

United Nations (1971). *Declaration of General and Special Rights of the Mentally Handicapped.* New York: UN Dept. of Social Affairs.

Other sources for further reading are available from:

Europe

Belgian Department of Cultural Affairs.
Netherlands Educational Care of the Handicapped Child, State Dept. of Education and Science.
Fact Sheets on Sweden, published by the Swedish Institute.

United States

U.S. Educational Commission.

Canada

Canadian High Commission.
Canadian Association for the Mentally Retarded.
Toronto Education Board; London Office of the Province of Quebec.

Australia

Royal Commission on Human Relationships 1977.
Australian Government Publishing Service.
The Subnormal Children's Welfare Association, New South Wales.
The Queensland Sub-normal Children's Welfare Association.
Australasian Express, January 6th, 1981.

CHAPTER 14

Implications for the Future

Ann and Michael Craft

The foregoing chapters have indicated what might lie ahead in the provision and development and services for mentally handicapped children, adolescents and adults. A number of key points have emerged:

(1) Sexuality is an Integral Part of the Human Condition

All humans are sexual beings with bodies that enjoy warmth, touch and pleasure; with strong impulses to forge intimate bonds; with inherent reproductive capacities; with genders which shape familial and social roles; with needs and drives that manifest themselves in many ways, both open and subtle. Mentally handicapped individuals have a right to channel their sexuality in ways which are normal for the society in which they live. They therefore have a right to the information and education which will enable them to do this.

(2) Social Education is Incomplete Without Sexual Education

Mentally handicapped individuals need sex education as a normal and natural part of social education. The situation at present is unsatisfactory for them and for us as parents and professionals. We are caught in a trap largely of our own making. At issue, stated and re-stated in many ways at every conference concerned with sexuality and mental handicap that we have attended, is this central point:

> Mentally handicapped children grow up and become men and women. Their socio-sexual behaviour does not accord with their physical maturity, and gives rise to problems for themselves and others.

A major factor in why this is so can be found in the distinction between 'puberty' and 'adolescence' (Murphy 1981). Puberty is a *biological* process which cannot be halted. It might, as is rumoured concerning young Olympic class swimmers and gymnasts, be

299

delayed by drugs, but eventually it happens. Voices break, pubic hair grows, breasts develop and menstruation begins, etc. Adolescence is the state or process of growing up, the time of transition between childhood and adulthood. It is a *social* process, as the individual develops his understanding of his own social and sexual identity. In many non-western societies the attainment of the biological, secondary sexual characteristics triggers the social process of becoming an adult. The 'adolescent' stage is usually accomplished in intensive training with special teachers over days, weeks or months in a place away from the community. The youngster leaves as a child, but returns as an adult, both in biological and social terms. In our society, we can and do deny adolescence and adulthood to mentally handicapped people. We cannot stop their physical maturity, but often, with the best of intentions, we stop or curtail their socio-sexual development. The result is persons who are physically adult, but who have the social status of children. Some would say that it is the mental handicap *per se* which inevitably gives rise to this state of affairs, but we would argue that while mental limitations do set parameters to social maturity, we are a long way from knowing what these parameters are. They will vary, not only with intellectual capabilities of individuals, but with upbringing, educational opportunities and environments. (We might draw a parallel here with literacy skills—the factor of intelligence is only one of many which determine whether an individual can read and write.)

(3) Sex Education is a Necessary Living Skill

Sex education does *not* simply refer to mechanics, nor simply to the physical act of sexual intercourse. Sex education touches upon relationships, social behaviour, gender identity, pleasure, caring, responsibility, hygiene, legality and morality. The amount and focus of information will vary according to individual capabilities.

We have seen how closely interlinked are social, health and sex education. We cannot afford to neglect any of the three, because in broad terms each has a vital part to play in the quality of life enjoyed (or endured) by mentally handicapped people. Each component, each 'brick' of knowledge and understanding, may be viewed as an adaptive living skill, the learning and practising of which are steps towards social maturity.

300

(4) Parental and Professional Responsibilities

Parents are potentially able to offer each other support and advice concerning the sexuality of their offspring. They may need initial assistance from mental handicap service professionals to set up self-help groups and specific in-puts of specialized information.

Parents may well consider themselves to be the best people to provide sex education to their children—indeed as we have seen, this education goes on informally within families from the moment a child is born. What, however, if there is a clash of principle concerning the provision of formal teaching between home and school, home and work centre, home and residential unit? Many parental objections are based on erroneous beliefs about what the school or unit is actually going to do. Tactful discussions and meetings, with a chance to view the teaching material to be used, may do much to dispel disquiet. Where mentally handicapped individuals are legally adult and parents object to their taking part in an education programme, again a tactful approach may relieve parental anxieties. The best course may be to start the programme with a few people whose parents are enthusiastic, then invite everyone to a review meeting after six or twelve months.

In the last resort, we believe professionals should consider very carefully to whom their responsibility lies—to the parent or to the mentally handicapped adult trainee or hostel resident.

(5) Counselling Services for Parents and Care Staff

Mental handicap care systems should be able to offer parents and residential staff access to a counselling service. This counselling should be given by professionals experienced in mental handicap, empathy being more important than any particular professional discipline. It should not simply be an *ad hoc* provision called into play by a 'problem' or 'crisis' although of course the counsellor has a vital role when these occur, but a regular service helping parents and care staff to look ahead to the future needs of particular mentally handicapped persons. As such, a counselling service works in tandem with sex education programmes for retarded individuals.

(6) Personal and Contraceptive Counselling Services for Mentally Handicapped Clients

Mentally handicapped persons may need special help in coping with the demands and responsibilities of intimate relationships. Pre- and post-marital counselling services should exist for couples wishing to marry, and for those experiencing problems with relationships or sexual expression.

At least one member of local or area family planning services might usefully specialize in mental and physical handicap, being aware of the particular difficulties either or both may impose on contraceptive counselling.

(7) The Need for Written Operational Policies on Sexual Expression to Guide Care Staff and Residents in Living Units

All residential units will find it of benefit to have agreed and written policies concerning the sexual behaviour of residents. These should not be a mere listing of rules, or worse, of prescriptions, but positive statements of rights and possibilities in the context of the law and mores of the state or country concerned. Administrative managers, care staff, domestic workers, and of course, residents themselves, should take part in the discussions. Having to formalize responses to behaviour and relationships so that a policy can be put down on paper is a very useful exercise. It is likely to show up many divergencies of opinion and belief (among mentally handicapped residents as well as staff) about what is and is not permissible, what ought or ought not to be allowed. Many an 'unwritten law' looks illogical, unfair or downright foolish when openly debated.

Policies should be reviewed regularly, perhaps once a year, so that new staff and new residents can voice opinions and are quite clear about everything.

(8) Professional Training Courses should Contain a Component on Sexuality and Mental Handicap

Teachers, trainers and care staff of mentally handicapped persons need specific help, education and training to respond consistently and positively to the sexual behaviour of those in their care. Such education should be included in pre-qualification courses, and have a place in in-service training programmes. Curriculum

302

re-adjustment may be necessary to allow time for lectures and discussions covering this vital area of human behaviour.

Until, as part of an overall service, we help parents and care staff to accept and respond positively to the sexuality of their mentally handicapped child or client, both in crisis and in calm; provide sex education and counselling as a matter of course in special schools and adult facilities; offer more normal living circumstances for those who cannot live at home; formulate guidelines with care staff; and listen carefully to what retarded people tell us about their sexual needs and feelings, we are not going to be much more than firemen dashing from one crisis to the next. Societies will always need their firemen, but it makes sense to place more and more emphasis on fire prevention. This is what our book has been about.

REFERENCES

Murphy, G.J. (1981). The Institutionalized Adolescent and the Ethics of Desexualition. In: Shore, D.A. and Gochros, H.L. (eds). *Sexual Problems of Adolescents in Institutions.* Springfield, Ill.: Charles C. Thomas.

...ation of Rights of the
...lly Handicapped – 31, 80,

vocabulary – 14, 65, 69, 92, 117, 127, 134, 138, 139

...isease – 16, 85, 110, 124–5, ...70

World Health Organization – 15, 110

Index

abortion – 16, 29, 63, 124, 225, 232–3, 250, 279, 288
adolescence – 19, 47, 99–101, 112, 118–19, 120, 131, 165–7, 205–6, 273, 274–5, 299–300 *see also* puberty
Adult Training Centre (ATC) – 101, 105, 106, 131, 144–5, 154, 291–2
adulthood – 78, 97, 101, 111, 119, 131, 139, 140, 145–6, 148, 168–74, 196, 239, 271, 291, 292, 300
assessment – 186–7
attitudes towards sexuality
 of mentally handicapped
  individuals – 8–9, 32, 214, 222–236, 268, 271, 272, 281–2, 302
 of parents – 4–5, 78–85, 96, 97, 100–1, 119–20
 of professionals – 5–8, 59–61, 74, 78–81, 96, 97, 100–1, 127, 135, 302
 of society – 3–4, 53, 110, 272, 288–9, 296
audiovisual resources – 16, 67, 76–7, 128, 133, 138, 148–9, 153–4, 159–60, 164, 167, 173–4, 179–80, 184
Australia – 295–6

behaviour modification – 10–11, 186–93, 199–211
Belgium – 294
birth control – 2, 5, 16, 18, 20, 26–31, 63, 85, 170, 214, 228, 241–53, 279–80, 281, 283, 291, 293
 Depo-provera – 27, 63, 245, 246–8
 IUD – 27, 63, 245, 247, 248–9
 other non-permanent measures – 27–8, 244–5
 pill – 27, 63, 232, 245–6
 vasectomy – 223, 232–4, 246, 249, 250, 264, 265–6 *see also* family planning service *and* sterilization
Blissymbolics – 295

Canada – 30–1, 75, 295
check lists of knowledge and skills – 188–91, 193–9, 204

children of mentally handicapped parents
conception – 67, 140, 141, 152 *see also* fertility *and* reproductive capacity
consent – 3, 26, 28, 29–31, 133, 140, 170–1, 209–10, 231–4, 251–2, 265–6
contraception *see* birth control *and* family planning service
counselling *see* sexual counselling
curricula – 16, 66, 69, 110, 121, 148–85, 291, 293, 295, 302–3
curriculum development – 110, 113–28

Denmark – 20, 21, 24, 110
Depo-provera *see* birth control
developing countries – 296–7
Down's syndrome – 9, 44, 49, 58, 296–7
dramatic play – 70–1, 90, 108, 128, 159, 176 *see also* role-play

Educables *see* ESN(M)
environment – 10, 17, 24, 39, 47–8, 108, 136, 209
ESN (M) – 4, 5, 8, 13, 15–16, 17–18, 66–7, 111, 112, 119, 127, 128–9
ESN (S) – 19, 66, 67–8, 111 *see also* severely handicapped individuals
ethical considerations – 208–10, 252
Eugenics movement – 1, 20
evaluation – 56, 128–9

family planning service – 26, 29, 241–4, 302 *see also* birth control
fertility – 9–10, 26, 248, 249, 250, 252, 264 *see also* reproductive capacity

group counselling – 137–44, 199–202, 255, 256–7, 266, 277–8, 295

health education – 110–30, 148–85, 194–8, 295, 300
heterosexual relationships – 62, 82, 200, 201–2, 217, 227, 241, 250
homosexuality – 16, 39, 40, 43, 46–8, 50, 62, 85, 124, 125, 140, 171, 172, 207

human body – 139, 149, 150–4, 194–5
hygiene – 111, 112, 161–4, 187, 196–7
  see also health education

ignorance *see* sexual knowledge
Institute for Sex Research – 39, 40
institutions *see* residential units
intrauterine device (IUD) *see* birth
  control

Jay Committee – 6

legal aspects – 30–1, 39, 50, 51, 86, 92,
  170–1, 292, 300, 302 *see also*
  consent *and* sexual offence.

marriage – 2, 3, 9, 19–22, 61, 62, 80,
  82, 83, 85, 93, 105, 119, 140, 141,
  172, 214, 230, 254–86, 287, 291,
  292, 294
masturbation – 6, 10, 19, 38, 40,
  42–3, 46, 49, 61, 73, 79, 85, 96,
  106, 108, 124, 125, 134, 135, 139,
  143, 164, 166, 202, 204–6, 226,
  272, 281
menopause – 172, 243–4
menstruation – 66, 73, 81, 85, 106,
  110, 126, 132, 139, 163, 166, 196,
  244, 247, 249, 250, 269
mentally handicapped parents – 61,
  62, 119, 140, 143, 172, 230–4
  competence – 23, 24–5, 32, 222–3,
    227, 230–1, 250, 262, 263, 292–3
  family size – 26
  risk of handicap in offspring – 2, 3,
    9, 20, 22–4, 25, 26, 105, 250, 262–3,
    279
  see also parenting
mildly handicapped individuals – 9,
  12, 19, 27, 29, 67, 96, 199, 213–40,
  241–9, 250, 254
Milwaukee Project – 25
Minnesota Institute of Human
  Genetics – 23
morals – 5, 31, 39, 127–8, 134, 138,
  149, 170–1, 300
multiply handicapped individuals – 18,
  90, 131–46
myths – 53, 57–8, 66, 84, 133, 213–14,
  281

Netherlands – 293–4
normality, models of – 38–41, 47

normalization – 1, 2, 6, 31, 63, 87–8,
  93, 213, 215, 253, 291, 297
Normalization Study – 215–17, 220,
  221

overprotection – 5–6, 44, 81, 83, 180,
  201, 281

parenting – 16, 32, 81, 119, 140, 143,
  172, 217, 219–21, 230–4, 239, 250,
  262–6, 271, 278–80, 291, 292–3,
  294 *see also* mentally handicapped
  parents
parents
  attitudes of – 4–5, 71, 78–85, 97,
    100–1
  concerns of – 72–3, 81–2, 99–101,
    144–5, 210, 249, 250–1, 258–60,
    280, 289
  counselling of – 78–94, 96, 274–6,
    281, 301
  part in sex education – 4–5, 13,
    18–19, 71, 111, 119–20, 301
  relationship with their child – 96–9
  support groups – 102–8, 145, 301
personal adjustment training –
  199–202
personal hygiene *see* hygiene
pill *see* birth control
PLISSIT model – 91–2, 273–7, 278
policy guidelines – 6–7, 32, 62, 74,
  85–9, 90–1, 134, 302, 303
postmarital counselling – 22, 78, 255,
  256–7, 276, 277–84, 302
premarital counselling – 78, 255,
  256–7, 276, 279–80, 302
privacy – 10, 101, 105, 106, 133, 134,
  138, 139, 166, 171, 205, 261, 272,
  288
professionals
  attitudes of – 5–8, 53, 56, 59–61, 97,
    134
  concerns of – 50, 51
  counselling of – 78–94, 96, 301
  as counsellors – 55–6, 62, 89–93
  training in sexuality – 6–8, 53–77,
    86, 302–3
  working with parents – 71–3, 301
psychosexual development – 4, 10,
  41–5, 46–7, 80, 214, 270–2
puberty – 4, 44, 118–19, 126, 165–7,
  288, 299–300 *see also* adolescence
  and sexual development

relationships – 4, 6, 16, 44, 61, 67, 80,
  118–19, 127, 133, 135, 136–7, 140,
  141, 143–4, 172, 175–80, 195, 211,
  217, 238, 242, 276, 295, 300, 302
reproductive capacity – 1, 2, 3, 9, 26,
  63, 217–21, 228, 238 *see also*
  fertility
residential units – 5, 6–8, 13, 38,
  39–40, 51, 133, 134–5, 145, 154,
  168, 198, 208–10, 241, 294, 302
  see also environment
rights of mentally handicapped
  people – 1, 2, 29, 58, 63, 74, 75,
  80, 88, 93, 105, 108, 110, 209,
  213–4, 238, 241, 279, 287, 291, 299,
  302
role play – 70, 73, 90, 107, 128, 137,
  139, 148, 157, 158, 166, 176, 177,
  178, 179, 193, 200, 202, 282

Scarborough method – 68
Schools Council Project: Health
  Education 5–13 – 112, 117–18
segregation – 3, 26, 47, 100–1
self-concept – 64, 91, 106–7, 115, 117,
  181–4, 194–5, 199–201
severely mentally handicapped
  individuals – 2, 9, 18–19, 46,
  67–8, 95–6, 106–8, 116, 129, 143,
  194, 199, 207–8, 241, 245, 249–50
  see also ESN (S)
sex education – 4, 5, 6, 7, 11, 13,
  14–19, 32, 57–8, 63–74, 80, 85, 90,
  95–6, 110–30, 131–46, 148–85, 214,
  227, 237–9, 241, 271, 281–3, 288–9,
  291–2, 294–5, 296, 299–300, 303
see also health education
of severely handicapped people –
  18–19, 67–8, 95–6, 106–8, 143,
  194–9, 207–8
sexual behaviour – 2, 3–4, 5, 6, 9,
  10–13, 15, 17, 39–52, 55, 62–3,
  82–3, 84, 125, 131, 133–8, 168, 170,
  191, 202–8, 243, 291, 302 *see also*
  sexuality
sexual counselling – 7, 50, 56, 61, 62,
  74, 78, 89–93, 126, 140, 237, 241–
  53, 254–86, 292–3, 301, 303
sexual development – 4, 9–10, 15, 81,
  139, 300 *see also* puberty
sexual deviation – 44, 45–8, 202

sexual dys[...]
  201–2[...]
  265, 2[...]
sexual exp[...]
  73, 8[...]
  182
sexual full[...]
  297
sexual ign[...]
sexual int[...]
  93, 10[...]
  300
sexual kno[...]
  58, 74[...]
  136, 1[...]
  214, 2[...]
sexual offe[...]
  170–1[...]
sexual opp[...]
sexual plea[...]
  227–3[...]
sexual pro[...]
  101–2[...]
  234–6[...]
  dysfu[...]
sexuality –[...]
  129, 1[...]
  254, 2[...]
  299 *se*[...]
  devel[...]
social cont[...]
  136–8[...]
socializatio[...]
  functi[...]
socio-sexu[...]
  14–15[...]
  136–8[...]
  270–2[...]
staff *see* pro[...]
sterilization[...]
  79, 100[...]
  237–9[...]
  264–6[...]
Sweden –[...]
  31, 110[...]

teacher pre[...]
teaching pr[...]
  148–85[...]
Trainables[...]
training tec[...]
  profess[...]